BIBLIOTHERAPY

IN THE

BRONX

BIBLIOTHERAPY
IN THE
BRONX

EMELY RUMBLE

Row House Publishing recognizes that the power of justice-centered storytelling isn't a phenomenon; it is essential for progress. We believe in equity and activism, and that books—and the culture around them—have the potential to transform the universal conversation around what it means to be human.

Part of honoring that conversation is protecting the intellectual property of authors. Reproducing any portion of this book (except for the use of short quotations for review purposes) without the expressed written permission of the copyright owner(s) is strictly prohibited. Submit all requests for usage to rights@rowhousepublishing.com.

Thank you for being an important part of the conversation and holding sacred the critical work of our authors.

Library of Congress Cataloging-in-Publication Data Available Upon Request
ISBN 978-1-955905-87-9 (HC)
ISBN 978-1-955905-88-6 (eBook)

Book design by Neuwirth & Associates, Inc.

Printed in the United States

Distributed by Simon & Schuster
First edition
10 9 8 7 6 5 4 3 2 1

CONTENTS

To my husband and best friend, Chad Rumble: Your boundless support and love mean the world to me. Thank you for believing in me and showing me the beauty of taking risks.

To my amazing children, Chaz Rumble and Quest Rumble: Your joy and curiosity inspire me to be better and dream bigger. You are the reason I strive to make a positive impact.

And to you, dear reader, for journeying with me and every other author who dared to share a truth with courage and conviction.

To "Readers Who Run with the Wolves"—you know who you are.

"Books are sometimes windows, offering views of worlds that may be real or imagined, familiar or strange. These windows are also sliding glass doors, and readers have only to walk through in imagination to become part of whatever world has been created or recreated by the author. When lighting conditions are just right, however, a window can also be a mirror. Literature transforms human experience and reflects it back to us, and in that reflection we can see our own lives and experiences as part of the larger human experience. Reading, then, becomes a means of self-affirmation, and readers often seek their mirrors in books."

—Dr. Rudine Sims Bishop

FOREWORD

I remember waiting for the 2 train to arrive at 72nd Street Station back in high school. If you've ever lived in the Boogie Down Bronx, you already know the reputation of the 2 and 5 lines—they take forever! There were eighteen train stops between 72nd Street and Pelham Parkway, but I didn't mind because I would use that time to read. I was a newbie to the Bronx as a teen, after my parents' tumultuous divorce, when I found myself triangulated as the oldest and parentified child. Reading, writing poetry, and music were my only outlets when I had no one to talk to. Reading was my escape. Writing was where I could channel my loneliness. Music was where I could journey with my tears without judgment.

I often saw myself in the characters of the books I read and would get lost daydreaming about different endings. Reading and poetry were the only places I felt safe enough to dream, and they also let me protect those dreams from an uncaring world. To think there was a time I couldn't afford to buy books in the Scholastic Book Fairs in elementary school saddens me, especially knowing how much books would save my life later in adolescence (and as a whole adult). Books would save me from depression during my parents' divorce and see me through some of the most painful moments in my life.

So, when I learned of Emely's bibliotherapy work, my heart rejoiced. It's important that you know that I first connected with her when she was amplifying my own book. When I, as a new author, was announcing the birth of my book baby, Em had already been speaking about the advance reader's copy (ARC) she received. On the day of my book launch, she dedicated an Instagram post to *The Pain We Carry*, set to the Spanish tune "Aguanilé." I will never forget the appreciation I felt that someone remembered, and she was that someone. Because, y'all, books have the power to bring people together. And it did here, for us—a testament to bibliotherapy fostering a sense of kinship and connection.

For as long as I can remember, the Bronx has had a bad reputation, saddled with many stereotypes. Racism, capitalism, and classism certainly play a role in these narratives, as the Bronx is home to many Latinx and Black communities. It is the borough that is most forgotten, and some have said it's the most dangerous and poverty-stricken, but many fail to see the deep medicine and vibrancy flowing through its veins. In *Bibliotherapy in the Bronx*, Emely reminds us of its profound influence. And as a Boricua who was raised in both the Lower East Side and the Bronx, I am proud.

You will see in this book that Em's bibliotherapy work is communal medicine and illuminates the healing that can be found in storytelling, not only for the Bronx but for the world. Her book serves as confirmation of the unwavering alchemical power of bibliotherapy. The stories of her clients, her own personal healing journey, and the rich history of bibliotherapy speak to the resilience of the human soul and the ability for us to deeply heal and transform through literature. We can find our stories, and those that resonate with us, and use them as a guide for our own reflections and inner-standing.

This book is potent, y'all. And needed. You will be transformed through the sacred power woven into these pages with Em's deep-rooted wisdom—from her vulnerable sharing to her bibliotherapy knowledge steeped in practice from the books she has read to both her lived and professional experience as a decolonial social worker centering marginalized and oppressed voices. She blesses us with bibliotherapeutic reflections that invite us to delve deeper into seeing ourselves and channeling the difficult emotions we try to hide (even from ourselves) using dope literature and prompts.

Emely reminds us that "books offer more than just lessons in personal growth; they also serve as roadmaps for societal change." As you take this literary journey, what emotional wounds are calling for your attention? Remember that healing yourself creates ripples of change and helps to heal our community, which helps to heal the world, because it's all connected. Books can serve as catalysts for change and liberation. May you find your sovereignty reading this book. May you taste liberation as you digest its words. Let it free you. Let it inspire you to dream again. Let it grieve with you. Let it love you. Let it heal you.

NATALIE Y. GUTIÉRREZ, LMFT
Author of *The Pain We Carry: Healing from Complex PTSD for People of Color*

WHAT YOU CAN EXPECT FROM THIS BOOK

This book explores the history of bibliotherapy and poetry therapy as modalities to support the treatment of mental health challenges. My goal is to share my experiences, both personal and professional, to make the case for the effectiveness of this modality. I won't talk much about who this modality isn't for. Instead, my focus is on speaking to readers whom this approach can support toward healing and self-actualizing. I hope this book will answer any questions you have about what bibliotherapy is and how it's implemented in therapy with a trained mental health professional. I also hope you're inspired to deepen your personal reading practice for your mental health.

In the chapters that follow, I will provide a brief overview of how literature has informed healing practice historically and in the present day. In Part 1, I explain what bibliotherapy is and how poetry therapy is a distinct intervention apart from using books. I include my personal story and journey to becoming a bibliotherapist. I also offer historical context and therapeutic insights from bibliotherapy practice that deepen our understanding of why books and the stories they carry are so integral to our healing. In Part 2, we do a deep dive into how reading unlocks mindfulness and increases self-awareness by helping us reflect and truly sit with our emotions from an embodied perspective. In Part 3, we specifically explore how books have contributed to our collective mental health. I focus on how the use of bibliotherapy nurtures our growth in community, with a focus on social justice and collective well-being. I conclude the book with a reminder of the importance of ease in our overall healing journey and how cultivating a love of literature helps us access softness.

At the end of each chapter are bibliotherapeutic reflections to help you consider what you've read in the context of your own life experience and reading practice. I firmly believe that what you reflect on in this book will illuminate who you are as a reader and why you gravitate to particular books and authors. You'll identify the ways your love of reading has made you feel seen and more connected to others.

Within each chapter's conclusion, you will find exercises designed to deepen your personal engagement with the content and help therapists seamlessly integrate the transformative power of bibliotherapy into their practices. As a therapist, I recognize the profound value in understanding how this book's access points can illuminate your identity as a reader while also providing therapeutic insights. We acknowledge that readers possess unique strengths, and as therapists, we can leverage these strengths to guide them on their healing journeys. Psychotherapy, inherently interpersonal, thrives on the client/therapist relationship. Recognizing that clients are already immersed in self-healing through their love of literature, we aim to build upon this intrinsic practice.

As lifelong learners, readers often seek answers within the pages of books, relying on research and facts. However, therapeutic progress requires engagement of the heart rather than solely the intellect. With our unique training, skilled therapists facilitate this transition from cognitive understanding to emotional connection. Emphasizing that therapy is not a purely analytical process, I encourage therapists to treat clients' books as integral elements of their support system. By engaging clients in discussions about literature that profoundly impacted them, therapists can help forge meaningful connections between the text and the client's emotions, blockages, desires, fears, and more. This approach transcends traditional therapeutic methods, fostering a deeper, more holistic healing experience for therapists and clients alike.

My hope is that with each exploration in this book, you will feel validated as a reader. So many of us grew up finding safety, comfort, and answers to life's greatest questions in books. Yet we were told to get our heads out of them. We were told to learn to deal with reality in family systems where keeping secrets was the norm, and the realities provided were only half-truths. We were even chastised for our love of reading, because we were seen as hiding from the world in our books. The loved ones who spoke to us this way did not understand, could not understand, that each time we read a book, we were better equipping ourselves to engage with the world. Through cultivating a love of reading, so many of us became clearer about our own station in life, the world at large, and the world our reading nook was a part of.

Maybe you, like me, grew up visiting the library for lack of a safe environment to be a kid. Maybe you grew up making regular trips to the bookstore to pick up books you couldn't find at school or that teachers and librarians told you were too mature for your age. Whatever the case, books have helped us survive and thrive. In books, we could be at home with ourselves, no matter what was happening around us. No matter the chaos, the unpredictable nature of our home life, the mood(s) of our parents or caregivers, the friends who betrayed us at school, the childhood crush who was mean to us, or the bully we worked so hard to try to avoid—books have always been there for us. Books have been our most constant, consistent friends. Through stories, we have been able to just be, with nothing else asked or required of us.

In a world where people are often treated like machines and not the divine beings we are, it's all too easy to forget to rest and play. Often, we forget how to feel; we forget to give our emotions about our life encounters a moment to rise to the surface where they can be noticed, felt, and expressed. The healing that needs to happen is in our ability to respect that we are human and we need to feel.

I'm so honored that you have chosen to read *Bibliotherapy in the Bronx*. May these pages edify you, teach you something new, and hold space for the reader in you to feel celebrated.

BIBLIOTHERAPY
IN THE
BRONX

INTRODUCTION

My journey into social work started in the Bronx in 2008. My first year as a student was at a day treatment facility for adults with schizophrenia. When I first received my placement, my field advisor called me to ensure that I understood the population I would be serving and felt comfortable with my assignment.

"Now, this is not usually an internship we'd give to a first-year," she said.

It wasn't the first time I had heard this sentiment. The director of field placements at Smith College School for Social Work had said the same thing to me several times. It was as if the administration at my school lacked confidence that I could handle it.

I told my field advisor I was more than fine with the assignment—I was excited. She didn't understand why I wasn't overwhelmed by the notion of working with such a high-need population as a first-year student. She didn't know how intimately acquainted I was with schizophrenia.

My maternal aunt, who babysat me, was diagnosed with paranoid schizophrenia. With this manifestation of schizophrenia, she rarely, if ever, left the house. While I was left in her care, all we did was watch soap operas and NBC News. Her favorite shows were *General Hospital* and anything on Univision. She often had *ideas of reference* about what the characters and newscasters were saying. Ideas of reference, in psychiatry, refer to someone mistakenly believing that ordinary events or things around them have special meanings or are directly related to them. For example, a person with ideas of reference might think a TV show is sending them secret messages or that strangers on the street are talking about them specifically, even when this isn't the case. My aunt would talk back to TV actors as if she were in the know about something she couldn't make me a part of. To keep me safe, she was always trying to manage the intrusive messages she was getting.

I remember one incident when we were watching one of her favorite soap operas, *All My Children*. Jack was speaking to his friend, who was teasing him about marrying Erica. Jack insisted that he wasn't the marrying kind and he would not be proposing. My aunt immediately decided we must start writing out the names of everyone who would want Jack and Erica married.

"Emely, we should make the wedding cards now," she said.

"What wedding cards, Titi?" I asked.

"Wedding cards for Jack and Erica so they can get married," she responded.

I was so confused. I didn't understand how making wedding cards was going to have any influence on Jack's decision not to get married. I also understood that my aunt might spiral into an episode if I didn't go along with her fantasy that it could help.

"Okay, what should I do?" I asked her.

Before I could finish my question, she was already grabbing some index cards from her desk and handing me a marker. I remember pretending to write, though, at the age of five, I had no idea how to spell. She smiled, relieved and pleased with herself for such a creative intervention. I smiled at how unpredictable her behavior could be and wondered if she was onto something that maybe I didn't understand because I was just a kid.

To my aunt, danger lurked everywhere, and everything, from a soap opera to a billboard, held a message or a sign. The weather report for the day could be a code for a conflict brewing in another country. An argument between fictitious lovers could put the fate of those characters in our hands, and we'd have to move quickly to act and change the course of events. Once, she made me rush to boil eggs so the voice speaking to her through the radio wouldn't show up at the door. I remember at first feeling like these were mini adventures that only she and I understood. I honestly felt honored that she chose to take me along for the ride. She trusted me, and I know she didn't trust many people.

According to *The Diagnostic and Statistical Manual of Mental Disorders, Fifth Edition* (DSM-5), schizophrenia is a chronic and severe mental disorder that affects how a person thinks, feels, and behaves. It is characterized by a combination of symptoms that can include hallucinations, delusions, disorganized thinking, disorganized speech, reduced emotional expression, and impaired social functioning. The exact cause of schizophrenia is unknown, but it is believed to involve a combination of genetic, environmental, and brain-chemistry factors. It typically emerges in late adolescence or early adulthood and can persist throughout a person's life. Symptoms of schizophrenia can vary in severity and may cause significant distress and impairment in daily functioning. Hallucinations, which are sensory experiences that are not based in reality, can involve seeing, hearing, or feeling things that others do not. Delusions are false beliefs that are not based in reality and can be bizarre or paranoid in nature. Disorganized thinking and speech can manifest as illogical thoughts and difficulties in organizing thoughts or expressing oneself coherently. My aunt's symptomatology was a broad range of all these manifestations.

In communities of color, where mental illness is often stigmatized or treated as a spiritual issue, it can be difficult to identify schizophrenia and seek treatment. Treatment for schizophrenia often involves a combination of antipsychotic medications, psychotherapy, and support services. With proper treatment and support, many individuals with schizophrenia can manage their symptoms, reduce the negative impact on their lives, and achieve a better quality of life. However, ongoing treatment and management are typically required to address the chronic nature of the disorder. This is why I was excited at the prospect of working at a Bronx day treatment facility, where a broad range of services made treatment available to the most vulnerable populations—which summoned memories of my aunt.

My understanding of mental illness came at an early age, but it wasn't until I reached kindergarten that I realized my aunt had a mental illness. As my babysitter, she would take me to the bus stop in the morning. This was when the difference between her behavior and that of the other parents and family members at the bus stop became strikingly clear. There was my aunt, speaking to herself aloud, in her robe, hair pointing up at the sky, undone, while the other parents stood far apart from us, warning their children to stay close to them. I remember thinking, *Why would anyone feel threatened by my sweet aunt? She'd never hurt anyone, especially not a child.* Now, don't get me wrong—there were many times I worried that she'd hurt herself, but she always treated me with such tenderness, I never questioned that I was safe when I was with her.

Aside from the fact that the reactions we received weren't aligned with my reality, the shame I felt and internalized during these bus-stop experiences was even more harmful because we lived in a predominantly white community in Meriden, Connecticut. Making sense of the laughs, stares, and judgment of others was a major contributor to my own racial trauma as a young girl navigating the white gaze.

As I grew older and developed more of an understanding of mental health issues and the way schizophrenia fragments the mind, I started to feel heartbroken about the way my family treated my aunt. She was believed to be possessed by demonic forces, and every time a pastor would visit to pray for her, I remember feeling her desire not to be touched. She would only let my grandmother lay hands on her. It was still hard to watch her in so much pain and to see the community around her try to pray it away instead of directly addressing her need for mental health treatment and support. I'm not sure when the official diagnosis of schizophrenia was given, but I know it most likely came after several crisis incidents at home that led to her being hospitalized, medicated, and treated.

The treatment of schizophrenia typically involves a comprehensive and multidimensional approach that combines medication, therapy, and support services. Antipsychotic medications are commonly prescribed to manage the positive symptoms of schizophrenia, including hallucinations and delusions. Additionally, psychotherapy can be beneficial in helping individuals develop coping strategies. Therapy aims to help individuals challenge distorted thoughts and improve social skills. In addition to medication and therapy, psychosocial interventions such as vocational rehabilitation, housing support, and social-skills training can promote independence and overall well-being. The day treatment facility where I would be interning provided this full range of services.

Due to the dynamic nature of schizophrenia, it is crucial that treatment plans are individualized and involve ongoing monitoring and collaboration between the individual, their health care team, and their support network to address the unique needs and goals of the person living with schizophrenia. I was excited to work with a team of social workers, psychologists, psychiatrists, and experts who'd dedicated their careers to working with a population that is too often misunderstood. The fact that most clients were BIPOC (Black, Indigenous, People of Color) excited me, as well.

When I arrived at the day treatment facility as a social work intern, I was immediately struck by one client, a European artist, who painted in the community room every morning. When I remarked on his gift, staff constantly warned me not to interact with him because of his borderline personality traits and the fact that, as a new intern, I was considered "fresh meat." I wasn't worried about the client taking advantage of my kindness or my innocence as a new social worker. Although I was a new student, I had been a student of life for many years. I felt confident about my role as a student social worker, and I knew I could hold my own.

When I was asked to start a therapy group to promote socialization among the clients, I immediately knew I would make it a poetry group. Poetry and literature are the two things I know best, and the creative gifts I was confident I could offer the program. I've been an avid reader my entire life, and my bachelor's degree was in English language and literature. I knew exactly how to use literature to help folks connect in communities. It's what helped me the most along my personal healing journey, particularly after the sudden death of my grandmother when I was fourteen. Literature helped me process grief, battle depression and suicidality, find my voice, and find my circle of support—my chosen family. I was certain it could do the same for the clients I was working with.

Initially, my supervisor wasn't too keen on my idea. In her mind, folks battling schizophrenia are too disorganized in their thinking and too separated from reality to enjoy poetry. "They either won't understand it, or they'll be too activated by language that's symbolic," she insisted. It immediately took me back to how my aunt would be activated by messages on the TV and radio. To my mind, if she was already receiving these messages, wouldn't something like a creative group that encouraged self-expression have helped her name what she was feeling? Maybe a poetry group would make my clients feel more connected and less alone. This could be a way to teach clients to trust again and to share their inner life and inner struggles. After all, this is the purpose of a socialization group.

The first poem I introduced to the group was the 1882 version of Walt Whitman's "Song of Myself." As a new social worker giving this modality a try, I felt comfortable reading this classic poem. I decided we would work with one stanza at a time so I could get a sense of what kind of poetry my clients would respond to. The poem begins:

> I Celebrate myself, and sing myself,
> And what I assume you shall assume,
> For every atom belonging to me as good belongs to you.

The opening of this poem was very soothing for some. One client's mother used to sing him to sleep, and he shared that he now sings the same song, "Sana, Sana," to himself to remember her. Another client shared that she was learning to celebrate her gains in treatment, although she still feels conflicted about taking so many pills and doesn't like the side effects they give her. At one point, a client who was activated started to bang his head on the wall, and a senior staff member walked in and escorted him out. I remember checking in with her afterward and having her tell me that he was "low functioning" and not appropriate for my group.

I felt the gut punch of forgetting to do an intake for every client beforehand. After that initial group session, I made it my mission to spend time interviewing each therapist in the program about their clients. I wanted to know the treatment goals they were working on and learn more about their unique presentation of schizophrenia. Once I had conducted this research, I could tailor my approach and create more structure for the group environment. I purchased notebooks from the 99-cent store for each client and used the next session to set ground rules, intentions for our time together, and ways of checking in with every client and their body to ensure they felt safe in the therapy room.

Once the group's ground rules were established, and we all agreed to them, the door stayed open for clients to exit and enter the room as they needed. We agreed to focus on one poem each week. We agreed that the final twenty minutes of group would be unstructured freewriting time. We also agreed that folks could decide to share or not share their writing with the rest of the group.

As I write this, it brings tears to my eyes, remembering how many clients decided to read their poetry aloud during our time together. And, my goodness, the poetry was beautiful. Clients were able to put their inner life on paper. The imagery they described provided a sensory experience that helped me and others to better understand the reality of their inner worlds and even their hallucinations and delusions. Their expression through creative writing also helped each of them to understand and cultivate relationships with one another. They understood more about each other's upbringing and the commonalities of the traumatic experiences they'd lived through.

Through sharing their stories, they could connect on a deeper interpersonal level. Socialization goal met!

In many ways, reading poetry, writing it, and sharing it in the community connected us all, and my clients kept returning to the group. New clients kept enrolling, and my poetry group became very popular at the program. I'm grateful to my supervisor, who, at the end of my internship, encouraged me to keep studying *bibliotherapy*, the use of literature to heal and teach new skills. She emboldened me to continue perfecting my craft. I didn't know at the time that bibliotherapy was a treatment modality one could be trained in. Whatever I was planning to do with my knowledge of literature and poetry, I was told to keep doing it. That's exactly what I did.

MY JOURNEY OF BIBLIOTHERAPY

At the time I am writing this, I am a licensed clinical social worker, school social worker, and early-childhood specialist in the Bronx, New York. Since 2008, I have worked with vulnerable, marginalized populations individually as well as in group and family environments. In 2020, I started my private therapy practice, Literapy NYC, in response to the impact the COVID-19 pandemic had on my career. This was the same year my son was diagnosed with autism, and I gave birth to my daughter. In the fight to obtain early-intervention services for my son while the world was in crisis, and to raise my daughter amid the threat of COVID, my practice became my opportunity to truly commit to my niche as a bibliotherapist—a psychotherapist specializing in the use of literature to heal. I believe in this modality because reading saved my life and helps me save lives every day.

Bibliotherapy is about more than reading for pleasure. It's about the way a love of reading activates us by allowing us to engage on an emotional and creative level with texts. It's about the way the texts we read empower us to fulfill our inherent potential. It's about how reading grants us respite from our self-consciousness in a way that allows us to be more at home with ourselves and in our bodies. This is huge, especially in marginalized communities, because rest can seem a lifetime away when you're overburdened by circumstances such as poverty, housing instability, racial trauma, and more.

For this reason, it feels important to state that, as an author and therapist, my work specifically takes a decolonial lens that centers the voices and experiences of BIPOC and other marginalized communities. As an African American, Puerto Rican, femme psychotherapist, I am committed to helping my people heal and reminding us that the best defense against a racist, sexist, homophobic, transphobic, xenophobic (we can go on and on) world is to educate ourselves. We read to understand the truth of the cultural-legacy burdens we carry. We read to connect to the truth of our history and to ways of ancestral healing and storytelling.

Bibliotherapy is not new. We have always used it, and so have our ancestors. Whether through the oral stories we pass down from generation to generation or through the written word, storytelling has always given us rich examples to internalize that provide grounding in who we are, where we've been, and the possibilities of where we can go.

My exploration into bibliotherapy has shaped my identity as a therapist and profoundly enriched my understanding of its transformative power in individual and community healing. Delving into the interplay between literature and therapeutic processes, I discovered that my journey as a bibliotherapist has equipped me with a nuanced approach to addressing the unique needs of my bibliophile clients. The process of selecting and engaging with literature has become a dynamic tool in fostering introspection, deeper empathy, and resilience. Through the lens of bibliotherapy, I've come to recognize the profound impact of narrative on both personal and collective well-being. This revelation has been instrumental in my work with clients from marginalized communities, where the healing potential of storytelling becomes a powerful means of navigating challenges rooted in systemic injustices. As I weave the threads of literature into the fabric of therapy, I find that it not only amplifies individual strengths but also serves as a communal tapestry, connecting us to our shared histories and possibilities. In essence, my exploration of bibliotherapy has made me a better therapist while illuminating the role a love of literature can play as a catalyst for both individual and collective healing.

PART ONE

THE HEALING HISTORY OF BIBLIOTHERAPY

CHAPTER 1

PAGES OF COURAGE AND SURVIVAL

"And even then, toxic stress is not only your painful present-day experiences (or your childhood trauma), but also the historical trauma of your ancestors still alive in your wounding, creating the long-lasting effects of intergenerational trauma in your family. And your wounds run deep."

—NATALIE GUTIÉRREZ, LMFT,
The Pain We Carry: Healing from Complex PTSD for People of Color

In this first chapter, we'll explore how books are trusted companions that support us when we can't rely on others. Books act like mirrors, giving comfort to those who feel broken. They teach us, give us strength, and help us identify and express our feelings. This journey looks closely at how stories can make us individually resilient and tie us together as a community.

Ready to roll with me and discover how books can turn us into storytellers, even when the world's playing hard to get with answers? Let's do this!

As a sixteen-year-old youth in foster care, I found comfort and understanding by reading Antwone Fisher's memoir, *Finding Fish*. This book became a guide, giving me strength to face unpredictable challenges. I identified with his journey in many ways, and his story helped validate my experience.

Reading a memoir based on the life of a young boy who survived childhood abandonment was my first experience with catharsis as a reader. As a foster kid, it was eye-opening to read about someone else dealing with the flashbacks, the uncertainty, and the powerlessness that comes with being an unassisted Black youth in America.

Fisher goes on a journey of self-discovery, but when he finally finds the answers he has been looking for, they do not provide the level of clarity and peace he is seeking. He soon realizes that the peace he seeks is a peace he must create for himself. The insight I gained from Fisher's story inspired me to remain hopeful at a time when I seriously considered ending my life. In this way, books are the most powerful mirrors, especially for those of us surrounded by broken glass.

Fisher's story gave me the insight I needed to learn that my suffering was not unique, and it was also survivable. While reading his book, I was preparing to become a legally emancipated minor. This was a difficult decision for me to make, as it required an appearance in court to terminate the parental rights of my biological parents. This was a milestone decision that was guided by the advice of my high school counselor. My counselor was a crystal-clear mirror for me and very honestly told me that the federal government would not offer me the financial aid I merited for college if I had working parents. At the time, I was living with my youth pastor and his family while caring for my own financial needs, working two jobs, and attending high school. What was reflected on paper was not the truth of my condition. Fisher's story gave me the insight to understand the choices I had to make and the strength I needed to step forward in making them.

My father never made it to the courtroom on the day of my emancipation hearing, and he never responded to the mandatory ad the court published in the newspaper. I don't even know if he knew I was fighting for his parental rights to be terminated. On the other hand, my mother showed up. I remember being floored because I didn't think she would make an appearance.

My mom stood in that courtroom and took it in. She accepted her mistakes and held herself accountable. She did not fight my right to seek emancipation. I will never forget when the judge asked her if she had any words; all she said was, "I love you, and I'm sorry." The judge told me she was proud of me and wished me luck on my life's journey. She said all this with eyes shining with visible tears that she fought to keep from falling.

My mother acknowledging the impact her abandonment had on me, however unintentional, was an insightful and affirming moment for me, too. Just like Fisher, I would learn to rebuild a more accurate mental representation of who I truly was after years of telling myself I was unwanted.

I remember walking back to the city bus stop after the court session ended. I was in shock that my legal freedom had been granted with ease. As I walked out of the courtroom, it started to rain. I felt like the sky was crying all the accumulated tears my heart had been holding.

There is a scene in *Finding Fish* that powerfully describes how I felt on the day of my emancipation in court:

Halfway home, the sky goes from dark gray to almost black and a loud thunder snap accompanies the first few raindrops that fall. Heavy, warm, big drops, they drench me in seconds, like an overturned bucket from the sky dumping just on my head. I reach my hands up and out, as if that can stop my getting wetter, and open my mouth, trying to swallow the downpour, till it finally hits me how funny it is, my trying to stop the rain.

Fisher speaks of surrender to the elements in life we cannot control. The rain can come at any moment. The sunshine can break through the clouds at any moment, too. It's the prophecy of the rainbow that the rain doesn't last forever.

Books provide us with the language we struggle to access when we are in survival mode, making our suffering a thing of beauty and nuance. As individuals from marginalized communities, we are always being measured against the lies of a culture poisoned by white supremacy. We are so used to being told what we do not have or cannot have access to. We are constantly assessed as deficient by systems never meant to serve us, just to keep us further oppressed.

We are always being told what we are *not*, without much focus on the very many unique and special things we *are*. We are fighters, healers, and seers. We are community caregivers, activists, leaders, and teachers. We are our ancestors' wildest dreams, even on our worst days and in the worst circumstances, because we are still standing despite the insurmountable challenges we have and continue to overcome.

THE GOALS OF BIBLIOTHERAPY

I am often asked if I think reading one book can resonate with a client in a way that meets all four of bibliotherapy's main goals:

1. Increase self-understanding by helping the client value their own personhood.
2. Improve the reality orientation of the client.
3. Improve the capacity to respond by enriching internal images and helping feelings about these images surface.
4. Increase awareness of interpersonal relationships.

My answer is always the same: It depends on the book, and it depends on the client. The art of reading the right book at the right time is about matching the client's needs with a book that addresses the themes they are dealing with. The art of book matching is finding a text that will answer the question the client is presently asking themselves.

One of the main things I have found that helps pair a client with the right book is to ensure that I've read the book first. When I've read the book, I develop an understanding of the story the book is telling, the central questions about life the book answers, and the literary devices the author used to tell the story. This helps me decide if a particular book would benefit a client. I like to refer to my reading intake process as *The Three Ps*: I consider the *presenting problem* the client is reporting; I consider their *preferences* as a reader; and then I provide a book *prescription* that will best address the client's needs.

The goal is always to help my client feel something. The goal is always to recommend trauma-informed literature that is honest about how life events change us. The goal is always to recommend literature that helps me teach this one lesson: When we allow ourselves the grace to be changed by life events, we can heal.

It would take years of my own therapy, healing, and unlearning to rewrite a truer narrative for myself around how I ended up in foster care. As the daughter of teen parents who was raised by my grandmother, there was no safety net. As a child, I did not and could not understand the why behind my father going into the military—why would he leave when all I wanted was his active presence? I did not and could not understand the why behind my mother not visiting. Why wouldn't she come to see me more often when her mother was raising me? It wasn't until my therapist asked me to consider my mother as a young parent at odds with her own mother, who would determine the motherhood role she could play, that I understood the tensions my mother was navigating. There were so many questions and not enough answers. And when we do not have someone to explain the whys, we end up creating narratives of our own, steeped in the bias, ignorance, and racism the world feeds us. Fisher's memoir was a prime example of a story that helped me question those false narratives at an early age. Little did I know that it would set the stage for the work I'd eventually do with clients.

MS. PARKINS, MY FIRST BIBLIOTHERAPIST

Ms. Parkins was my first-grade teacher and an educator I will never forget. In her classroom, we made stories come to life using music, dramatic play, puppet shows, and more. In her classroom, books became portals that helped me make connections between my chaotic home life, the confusing events I was observing, the questions I had that no one would answer, and the greater world at large.

When using bibliotherapy with children and youth, follow-up activities also encourage the use of other developmental skills, including motor skills, cognitive abilities, and language skills. Teachers can incorporate the use of activities to make reading meaningful.

I will never forget how Ms. Parkins used *Strega Nona*, by Tomie dePaola, to teach us the foundational importance of trust in relationships. Strega Nona is a witch who uses her magic to make and multiply her pasta. When she asks her neighbor, Anthony, to watch over her pasta while she runs an errand, she thinks she can trust him. When he messes with her pasta and mixes up her spell, and the pasta overflows from the pot into town, he puts her at risk. As a result, she sets boundaries with him and kicks him out of her home. It was the first lesson I learned about trust and the first time I fell in love with a book. Tomie dePaola was born in Meriden, Connecticut, just like I was—and here he was, writing a book about a witch, a role I always wondered about as a young girl who comes from a lineage of healers.

Strega Nona was an older woman, just like my abuela. She cared for her community, and she hid her gifts for fear of the consequences, just like my abuela. I did not need to know the full truth of my grandmother's story to quickly understand that honoring our ancestral spirituality comes at a cost. My young mind understood that Strega Nona kicked Anthony out of her home for his lack of awareness, which would have gotten her persecuted. In my mind's eye, I always wondered why she, rather than he, would be persecuted. Reading this story in the first grade helped me make connections between my own family's ancestry, women's history, and the world at large.

Strega Nona had deep meaning in my life, as the granddaughter of a healer. My abuela never spoke with me directly about her indigenous Taino spirituality. By the time I was born, my abuela was a devout Seventh-day Adventist. I once overheard my mother speak about how my abuela would cure her colds with natural remedies and prayers. My grandmother used to dress in all white. In many Latinx spiritual traditions, the wearing of white holds profound significance deeply rooted in historical and cultural contexts. This practice, often associated with Santería, Candomblé, and other syncretic Afro-Caribbean religions, symbolizes purity, peace, and spiritual cleansing. Historical context reveals that during the transatlantic slave trade, enslaved African people in the Americas were forced to convert to Christianity by their European captors. In response, they merged their ancestral African beliefs with Catholicism, creating syncretic faiths. White clothing is believed to appease the orishas (spirits or deities) and provide a neutral canvas for the practitioner's connection with the divine. It signifies spiritual rebirth and the shedding of negative energies, allowing individuals to commune with their deities and ancestors.

My abuela had a keen intuition and could predict things others couldn't. She would look at the sky and know when a storm was on its way. She would catch the scent of a woman and know the woman was pregnant. The first time I asked her about ancestral spiritual practices was the last time I asked. "Nosotros somos cristianos," she proclaimed—we are Christians. And that was the end of the conversation. In Ms. Parkins' classroom, the conversation could continue through literature and all the activities she built around stories.

MAKING READING MEANINGFUL:
DEVELOPMENTAL BIBLIOTHERAPY

I still remember the feeling I had when Ms. Parkins asked us to put on a play based on *Strega Nona*. Cast in the role of Strega Nona, I went all out with my outfit, wearing a wig and apron. I got creative with materials, and my friends and I made fake spaghetti using Play-Doh. We had so much fun, and Ms. Parkins was so entertained by the way we each experienced and chose to retell the story.

In developmental bibliotherapy, where the aim is to teach new skills or a moral lesson, a young person's use of imagination helps provide a learning experience that will make the subject material of the literature meaningful and applicable to their own lives. Follow-up activities allow children to exercise self-reflection and use their creativity to share impressions from the story. In Ms. Parkins' classroom, I found a home in literature and gained the vital skill of interpreting my life through a broader lens, which became a vehicle for self-empowerment and self-discovery at a young age.

BIBLIOTHERAPY

THE PROCESS IN PRACTICE USING
STREGA NONA A BOOK BY TOMIE DEPAOLA

1. We're exploring the theme of trust. Strega Nona trusts Big Anthony and leaves her home in his care.

2. Big Anthony breaks her trust by touching her pasta. Question for the reader: Do you identify most with Big Anthony or Strega Nona?

3. Deeper exploration of trust. Other questions we can ask the reader:
   - How does it feel when a friend breaks our trust?
   - When we break a friends trust, how might they feel?

4. Adult-led discussion and insights can be gained. Consider asking the following:
   - Who are some people you trust and why do you trust them?

5. This is when universalization of insights is made. What we may come to understand from this title:
   - Trust is earned and can be broken.
   - If trust is broken, it must actively be repaired for the relationship to heal.

DEVELOPMENTAL BIBLIOTHERAPY WITH
RUBY FINDS A WORRY BY TOM PERCIVAL

One of my favorite reading selections for developmental bibliotherapy with children who struggle with anxiety is *Ruby Finds a Worry* by Tom Percival. As a child, I struggled with intense anxiety, and this is a book I wish I'd had when I was navigating that early part of my development.

This book provides a meaningful opportunity to incorporate both bibliotherapy and narrative therapy (more on narrative therapy later) into my work. Ruby is a child who is followed around by a yellow cloud—her worry. We travel with Ruby through her day and witness how the cloud grows and affects her ability to be in the present moment. Only when she meets another child who is also followed by a cloud does she realize that she is not alone and that other children have similar worries.

By forging a connection with another child who relates to her, Ruby is less consumed by the cloud of her worry. As a result, the worry grows smaller and begins to affect her less. The moral of the story is that worry is a part of life. Worry will always be there, but worry doesn't have to be the size of a monster. We can minimize worry through connections with others and enjoy the joyful parts of life despite our anxiety.

BIBLIOTHERAPY IN PRACTICE

3 STEPS TO EXTERNALIZING THE PROBLEM USING
RUBY FINDS A WORRY BY TOM PERCIVAL USING
PRACTICES FORWARDED BY STEVE GADDIS

1. Identify the problem:
   - What is the problem you wanted to talk about?

2. Name the problem:
   - You are calling the problem X.
   - Is this a name that "fits" for you and your experience?

- If not, what other name might you give it?

3. Deconstruct the relationship to the problem:
   - When did X enter your life?
   - What kind of relationship do you have with X?
   - How does X get you to think about yourself?
   - What are X's primary messages for you?
   - What does it want for your connections to other people?

The early childhood educator George H. Whipple wrote extensively about how these types of illustrations in children's literature can help facilitate the bibliotherapeutic process and teach emotional literacy. In *Ruby Finds a Worry*, the illustrated worry, as depicted by a growing cloud, is central to teaching children something necessary and valuable: We are not the sum of our problems. Ruby learns that a problem is separate from the essence of her being. By acknowledging the worry that stalks her and identifying it as a problem, Ruby can consider her relationship to the problem and, with assistance, find creative solutions to cope with and reduce her worry.

Creating a positive and inclusive learning environment in the classroom and promoting literacy as an enjoyable experience is also a preventative measure to reduce the possibility of literacy trauma. Literacy trauma refers to negative psychological and emotional experiences that we may endure due to difficulties or challenges in acquiring literacy skills. It can result from various factors, such as learning disabilities, inadequate educational resources or support, social and cultural barriers, or traumatic experiences related to reading and writing. When children and young people see themselves and their realities reflected in literature, they can engage in enjoyable reading experiences. Developmental bibliotherapy allows children to discover the joy of reading, or being read to, for pleasure, free from the pressures of academic or performance expectations. Damn, I miss first grade!

THE POWER OF NONFICTION AND FICTION IN BIBLIOTHERAPY

Now that we've explored healing and the developmental potential of bibliotherapy in its application to early childhood, let's discuss the distinctive roles of nonfiction and fiction in supporting treatment goals for people of all ages. Understanding when and how to incorporate each genre into therapy can significantly enhance the therapeutic process. I love this about books!

Nonfiction: Providing Context and Psychoeducation

Nonfiction books serve as valuable resources, offering a wealth of information, context, and psychoeducation (the process of educating patients and their loved ones to better understand a specific mental health condition). They can empower readers by providing concrete knowledge about our condition, experiences, and struggles. Here are a few ways nonfiction can be beneficial:

Historical Context: Many mental health issues have historical roots, and understanding this context can help clients make sense of their experiences.

Joy DeGruy is a renowned clinical psychologist, researcher, educator, and author known for her groundbreaking work on the enduring impacts of slavery and racism on African Americans. Her influential book, *Post Traumatic Slave Syndrome*, offers a profound exploration of the intergenerational trauma that African Americans continue to grapple with in the present day. This is one of my favorite nonfiction books to recommend in bibliotherapy because DeGruy provides a comprehensive analysis of how the legacy of slavery reverberates through generations, affecting individuals and entire family lineages.

DeGruy meticulously examines the psychological and emotional scars that have been passed down through the centuries. Recognizing the significance of these inherited wounds, we can begin to heal, cultivate resilience, and work toward breaking the cycle of trauma, ultimately paving the way for a brighter and more empowered future. *Post Traumatic Slave Syndrome* serves as a vital resource for fostering awareness, healing, and empowerment within African American communities, encouraging a dialogue on the lasting effects of slavery and the path toward recovery from racial trauma.

Psychoeducation: Nonfiction books often present expert insights, coping strategies, and evidence-based treatments.

Stephanie Foo is an author and podcast producer known for her candid storytelling and profound insights into mental health and trauma. Her book *What My Bones Know: A Memoir of Healing from Complex Trauma* is a poignant and illuminating exploration of her journey through complex post-traumatic stress disorder (C-PTSD).

In this essential memoir, Foo courageously shares her own experiences, making C-PTSD relatable and understandable for readers. Through her narrative, she educates readers about the complexities of C-PTSD while also offering a deeply empathetic and insightful perspective on its emotional toll and consequences. Foo's book acts as a guiding light for individuals seeking to navigate their own path toward healing and self-discovery, encouraging them to confront their traumas and embark on a journey of self-restoration and empowerment.

Information for Growth: Self-help and personal-development books can offer practical guidance for growth and self-improvement.

James Clear is a prominent author and expert in the field of habit formation and personal development. His book *Atomic Habits* has had a profound impact on readers worldwide, offering a scaffolded approach to building positive habits and fostering overall well-being.

In *Atomic Habits*, Clear combines scientific research with practical insights to help readers grasp the mechanics of habit formation. He explains how tiny, consistent changes—atomic habits—can lead to significant and lasting personal growth. The book serves as a comprehensive guide, teaching readers how to break free from destructive habits and cultivate new, beneficial ones. It empowers readers with the knowledge and strategies needed to create a healthier and more fulfilling lifestyle, focusing on physical, mental, and emotional well-being.

Fiction: Experiencing Emotional Catharsis

Fiction offers a unique and immersive way for clients to explore emotions and experiences through the lens of fictional characters. Fiction allows readers to engage with complex feelings and situations in a safe and controlled environment by providing a window into characters' life experiences. Here's how fiction can be a powerful tool.

Emotional Catharsis: Fictional narratives often mirror real-life struggles and emotions, enabling readers to identify with characters' experiences and achieve emotional catharsis.

Emotional catharsis may be more accessible and beneficial through fiction rather than nonfiction for several reasons. Fiction provides a level of narrative distance, allowing readers to engage with emotions without feeling immediately connected to real-life experiences. The symbolic representation in fictional stories enables readers to relate to emotional content without confronting direct details. The escapism offered by fictional worlds creates a safe space for emotional exploration, free from judgment. Creative expression in fiction uses language and literary devices in bold ways, enhancing emotional impact and facilitating a unique perspective that becomes the reader's own. Controlled environments in fictional narratives allow individuals to navigate emotions at their own pace, fostering a sense of control. With multiple perspectives and universal themes, fiction can offer a diverse and relatable platform for emotional exploration, providing comfort and validation to those who share similar struggles or triumphs.

Andrea Beatriz Arango is an author whose work tackles important issues with sensitivity and authenticity. Arango's work offers a space for readers to identify with characters' experiences, achieve emotional catharsis, and find validation in acknowledging their own journeys. Nobody can write the voice of a middle-grade reader like Arango, in my opinion!

Her book *Iveliz Explains It All* reflects the experience of a Puerto Rican middle school–aged girl while also shedding light on the complexities of therapy and medication. Readers follow the journey of Iveliz, a young girl navigating the challenges of mental illness and therapy while facing the potential judgment of her religious grandmother. The book offers a rare glimpse into the life of a character who is unapologetically struggling to accept help and take medication, providing much-needed representation for young readers who share similar struggles.

The story also explores Iveliz's process of adjusting to the sudden loss of her father. This heart-wrenching experience is sure to resonate with those who have faced similar tragedies. By portraying the mother/daughter relationship and the shared experience of grief, the book authentically mirrors real-life struggles and emotions, making it relatable and emotionally cathartic. *Iveliz Explains It All* stands as a testament to the power of literature to help individuals feel seen and understood, especially when grappling with mental illness and family dynamics that may challenge their pursuit of healing and well-being.

Increased Awareness: Fictional stories encourage empathy and a broader perspective, helping clients gain insight into their own lives from a safe distance.

Kacen Callender is a critically acclaimed author celebrated for their powerful storytelling and contributions to the LGBTQ+ literary landscape. Their book *Felix Ever After* provides an especially important voice and representation for adolescent readers who identify as transgender. *Felix Ever After* honors the trans experience and delves into the complexities of self-identity, love, and acceptance. In a world where trans kids face disproportionately high rates of suicide, homelessness, and discrimination, this book offers much-needed comfort and validation. *Felix Ever After* is a valuable resource for parents and caregivers, equipping them with the tools and language to support their trans children.

Reality Orientation: While fiction isn't fact, it can help clients explore and navigate their own realities.

Elizabeth Acevedo is celebrated for her powerful narratives and dynamic storytelling. Her novel *The Poet X* resonates deeply with the youth I counsel and audiences of all ages, emphasizing the importance of creative expression and personal growth. In this book, Acevedo introduces us to Xiomara, a young girl navigating the challenges of growing up in a religious environment that often suppresses her creative spirit. The book beautifully illustrates the struggle many young people face in reconciling their personal passions with the expectations of their communities.

Through Xiomara's journey, readers are encouraged to honor their right to creative expression and self-discovery, even in the face of cultural or religious constraints. Acevedo's poetic prose and relatable characters provide a compelling example of how art can be a powerful tool for self-empowerment and growth. *The Poet X* helps young readers navigate their own realities and encourages them to embrace their unique voices and stories. Acevedo's novel serves as a vital reminder that creative expression is a universal right and a potent means of self-discovery.

CHOOSING THE RIGHT BOOK

As you've seen, both fiction and nonfiction are valuable tools in bibliotherapy, offering distinct approaches to supporting clients' treatment goals. By understanding each client's needs and preferences, therapists can select the right book to elicit emotions, provide information, increase awareness, and aid in reality orientation. The careful selection of the books we read throughout the therapeutic journey is an effective method for personal growth and healing.

How do we know what kind of book to prescribe to a client? Selecting the appropriate book for a client truly depends on their treatment goals, reading preferences, and therapeutic needs.

We start by conducting an intake to get to know our clients as readers. This helps us make a book match that will emotionally and psychologically benefit the work being done in the therapy room. In other words, we want to get at the heart of what a book prescription will do to enhance other aspects of the work.

If you're a therapist, consider the question the client is facing and then recommend a book that answers that question in the client's preferred genre, with the intersectionality of the client's identity in mind. Understanding the client's preferences as a reader involves thoughtful consideration of a few important things. First, it's best to consider if the client will benefit most from choosing their own reading material, having the therapist recommend a text, engaging in expressive writing as an intervention, or a combination. Second, the therapist should consider the client's life circumstances and evaluate how the chosen literature aligns with their current state and readiness for self-reflection. Last, assessing the client's receptivity to the style of writing, genre, format, or mode of representation is important in tailoring the bibliotherapeutic approach to their unique preferences and comfort.

When we read literature that we connect with at the right time (which is always when we need it most), we can allow our emotions to surface so we can view ourselves more clearly. We allow the emotions where our wounds reside to be felt, witnessed, and heard while bringing them into our conscious awareness. As I always tell my clients, "You must be able to admit the truth to yourself before you can say it to me. You have to be able to locate the wound." Once we identify the location of the wound, we can treat it. This is how healing happens.

Beyond the therapeutic selection of books to heal, we can also reflect on the ways the books we've always loved and return to often serve as mental health anchors. The books we enjoy reading and rereading speak to something inside us in a way we should pay attention to.

In the bibliotherapeutic reflection that follows, my colleague, Loren Cahill, reflects on how Kiese Laymon's book *Long Division* has served as a source of guidance and affirmation for her. By integrating the text into the affirmations she practices daily, she is reminded of revision's crucial role in our ability to heal and honor our experiences.

BIBLIOTHERAPEUTIC REFLECTION, BY LOREN CAHILL:

Kiese Laymon is one of the best authors of all time. In my third read of *Long Division*, the themes of time travel, grief, loss, love, and self-possession healed my insides in ways I didn't know were possible.

One simple reading ritual that grounds me on my toughest days is answering for myself Laymon's True/False quiz in *Long Division*, which his two protagonists, Baize and Citoyen, complete. I typed up the blank quiz and placed it on my altar. I often read the prompts aloud and shout out my revised answers. They often change. Maybe they are supposed to, if we are doing the hard work of reckoning. On the days when my courage sits alongside my creativity, I write short-answer responses to each. My submission below is one of my favorite attempts at this exercise. I hope my reflections support you in your own bibliotherapy practice.

True or False (or Maybe Fill in the Blank …)

Name: Loren S. Cahill
1. *Desperation will make a villain out of you.* <u>TRUE</u>
   But breakdowns can be breakthroughs. You will slowly come to learn how to make a discipline out of your dreams.

2. *Only a fool would not travel through time and change their past if they could.* <u>TRUE</u>

The transformation of regret to recommitment is the best way to create a new timeline.

3. You were brought to this country with the expectation of life, liberty, and the pursuit of happiness.   <u>FALSE</u>
    But even the progeny of the master's tools can be reverse-engineered into a freedom fighter.

4. If you push yourself hard in the direction of freedom, compassion, and excellence you will recover.   <u>FALSE</u>
    Hardness is no longer the goal. Find the spiritual project in your pursuit of softness.

5. Loving someone and loving how they make you feel are the same thing.   <u>FALSE</u>
    True love is revision. Run far and fast away from people who are committed to their/your first draft.

6. Only those who can read, write, and love can move back and forward through time.   <u>TRUE</u>
    Your creative process is the formula for time travel. Tell everyone else that you also want to get free.

7. There are undergrounds to the past and future for every human being on earth.   <u>TRUE</u>
    The subaltern will remind you of the other four senses. Believe beyond what you can see in front of you.

8. If you haven't read, written, or listened to something at least three times, you have never really read, written, or listened.   <u>TRUE</u>
    Find the time and remember that it can bend for work as holy as this.

9. *Past, present, and future exist within you and you change them by changing the way you live your life.*   <u>TRUE</u>
   Your body contains a whole loveline. Why are you afraid?

10. *You are special.*   <u>TRUE</u>
    The world is waiting for you to change it in a dot-dot-dot special way.

Bonus: Write a question you've been afraid to ask. What is that question?

Kiese Laymon's work reminds me to avoid the pitfalls of "slow death" and try my best never to become a "monster" or "a human being that I claim to despise" by abdicating my accountability to that which I love. *Long Division* reminds me in my darkest moments that "something more came before [this] and something more is coming after it." This book reminds me to hold space for myself. It also taught me that my imagination, honesty, and pen are my lifesaving equipment. If you have not found your way to *Long Division*, I hope my words lead you there. I also hope that if this special book does not speak to your soul, you find another that holds you together so you can pull a few lines to affirm yourself during the moments you need those reminders most.

CHAPTER 2

THE ORIGINS OF BIBLIOTHERAPY AND THE ROLE OF LIBRARIANSHIP

"Libraries and books encourage reflective thought. We cannot delegate the whole burden of returning balance to our lives to classes and therapeutic groups. A book creates a mindfulness class of one."

—ANDREW PETTEGREE AND ARTHUR DER WEDUWEN,
The Library: A Fragile History

In ancient Egypt, it was understood that books were medicine and that language, whether through words or images, communicated our deepest needs, feelings, thoughts, and desires. In ancient Greece and Rome, many philosophers made it their mission to write about the healing power of books and the importance of educating the mind, heart, and spirit through a love of literature. The Stoics believed we could control our moods and our thoughts. A love of literature was considered an important mechanism to help us do that. Libraries have ancient origins, dating back to the libraries of ancient Mesopotamia and Egypt. However, the modern concept of public libraries emerged during the Enlightenment in the seventeenth century, reflecting a shift toward promoting knowledge-sharing and education as essential components of a democratic society.

As early as 1272 CE, the Al-Mansuri Hospital in Cairo prescribed readings from the Qur'an as part of its medical treatment to patients.

The ancients understood that a love of reading illuminates the truth of who we are, the history of our ancestry, and the possibilities that exist for creating the life we want, even if we've never seen it modeled before. A love of reading connects us to home, whether it is the home that resides within each of us, the home we are working to create, or the one we've left and long to reside in once again. Building on this foundation, the role of literature in coping with challenging circumstances, such as wartime, takes center stage in this chapter.

THE LIBRARY WAR SERVICE

Books have long been used in treating war veterans who have navigated the experience of being away from home in foreign lands. The Library War Service (LWS) was a World War I initiative to provide library services and reading materials to soldiers and military personnel. It was organized by the American Library Association (ALA) and operated from 1917 to 1920. The ALA issued the first official definition of bibliotherapy in 1966: "The use of selected reading materials as therapeutic adjuvants in medicine and psychiatry; also guidance in the solution of personal problems through directed reading." The LWS recognized the importance of providing intellectual and recreational resources to soldiers to alleviate boredom and support their morale and well-being during their service. Books were a portal back to familiarity and the comfort of family.

The LWS also recruited and trained librarians to serve as camp librarians who would oversee the organization and operation of libraries within military installations. These librarians aided soldiers in assessing and selecting reading materials, organized book clubs and discussion groups, and facilitated educational and recreational activities. After WWI, the LWS ceased its operations. However, the ALA continued to support library services for military personnel during conflicts such as WWII and subsequent wars. These efforts have taken different forms over the years, with initiatives like the ALA's United Service Organizations (USO) Library Program and collaboration with military libraries. The ALA continues to be involved in supporting veterans' services and providing resources for military families.

A pamphlet printed by the ALA, titled *Library War Service*, explores the service of bibliotherapy, providing books as medicine, library reference service, and teaching illiterate soldiers. Although the ALA expanded on the definition of bibliotherapy in 1966, Samuel McChord Crothers coined the term *bibliotherapy* in 1916. During WWI, Crothers wrote many articles and was well known for his humor and intellect as a minister and essayist. One of his most popular articles was about his friend Bagster, who ran what he called a "Literary Clinic" to meet the needs of those struggling with their mental health but unable to afford treatment. The following guidance on what the soldiers were reading demonstrates the range of reasons for borrowing books:

> Soldiers read more than people in civil life, partly because they are away from home and need diversion, and partly because they are preparing themselves for a profession which is entirely new to them. In most camps the call for fiction is a little below fifty percent. It is rarely above that figure. The soldier reads to learn even more than he reads for recreation.

Trauma can profoundly affect our ability to fully integrate and process certain experiences or aspects of ourselves. War trauma disrupts one's sense of safety, coherence, and connection and leads to various psychological and emotional challenges. The LWS recognized the importance of supporting soldiers' well-being and acknowledged the value of reading and library services in a wartime context. Soldiers battling depression, addiction, PTSD, and other afflictions would be able to check out a book for connection, pleasure, or simply an escape from the day-to-day reality of being at war.

SADIE PETERSON DELANEY,
THE GODMOTHER OF BIBLIOTHERAPY

Discovering the pioneering work of Sadie Peterson Delaney (1889–1958) in the field of bibliotherapy was a revelatory experience for me as a bibliotherapist and a Black woman. A librarian and social worker, Delaney's contributions have reshaped the use of bibliotherapy through the lens of her unique intersectionality. Her work has had a profoundly empowering impact on those, like myself, who have only become more recently familiar with her groundbreaking legacy.

In her article "The Place of Bibliotherapy in a Hospital," Delaney wrote:

> The World War left a vast number of men broken in body and spirit and suffering from various disabilities. Some must put in long periods of hospitalization and in an effort to aid in their recovery, the Veterans Administration Hospital Libraries bridge the gap between the hospital and the outside world; aiding them in their adjustment to present conditions and fostering hope for a future.

Delaney would go on to be acknowledged for her many achievements as a librarian of distinction in the New York Public Library System and the Veterans Administration Hospital at Tuskegee, Alabama. She started her career as a social worker at Miss McGovern's School of Social Work in Poughkeepsie, New York, where she was raised. At thirty, she began working at the 135th Street branch of the New York City library system, the Schomburg Center for Research in Black Culture. In 1923, she became the head librarian at the Veterans Administration Hospital in Tuskegee, where she organized the hospital's library.

Delaney was a pioneer in group therapy and bibliotherapy for the mentally ill and received international acclaim for her volunteer work with blind people and delinquent youth. She trained librarians from other countries, including South Africa. Her work with the

Library of Congress and the ALA's Committee on Work With the Blind is a testament to her commitment as an active civic leader, librarian, and social worker. Today, the Sadie Peterson Delaney African Roots Branch Library in Poughkeepsie is named in her honor. On the day of the Atlanta University commencement banquet and the same evening she received her honorary doctorate, Delaney said:

> Were I a poet tonight, I might put my emotions in verse; were I an artist, I would paint a picture and title it "for those who serve"; were I a singer, I would sing "Hallelujah"; but am only a servant and can say, this is my finest hour.

This is my finest hour. That hits powerfully as a Black woman. Delaney's finest hour was being able to serve and being acknowledged for her service and legacy.

In a world where Black women's work is often undervalued, underappreciated, and frequently appropriated or straight-up stolen, reading these words is a reminder to all of us everywhere of centering our purpose over our need to be seen. Delaney didn't do the work she did because she wanted to be hailed as a leader. She did it because she wanted to help her people—her community—to heal. As a social worker, Black librarian, and community activist, she used her love and knowledge of literature to show the world that healing through the creative and expressive arts is possible.

There are many other important figures in Black librarianship whom I came to learn about in my research. In the rich tapestry of bibliotherapy, we must acknowledge and celebrate the indispensable role of Black librarians. Their significance extends far beyond the library walls; it is woven into the very fabric of American history. In a time when Jim Crow laws sought to segregate and subjugate, Black librarians became beacons of hope in a sea of adversity, establishing their own libraries, no matter how underfunded or underresourced. These libraries, often under constant threat, became sanctuaries of knowledge and cultural preservation where people living in marginalized and disenfranchised communities could access literature that enriched their lives, empowered their education, and allowed for the pure joy of literary escapism and bookish joy.

The legacy of Black librarianship is a testament to resilience, determination, and unwavering commitment despite persecution. There was a time when our ancestors were not allowed the right to learn to read and could be killed for it. Thanks to the dedicated efforts of Black librarians historically (and in the present day), Black literature became readily accessible, offering mirrors for readers to see ourselves reflected in stories. This was not merely a luxury; it was life-giving and life-sustaining for Black people. The tireless work of Black librarians transcends the confines of bookshelves, embodying a profound cultural and historical force that continues to shape our world today.

ON THE SHOULDERS OF GIANTS

As an African American, Puerto Rican bibliotherapist with a profound understanding of the labor of love that is Black librarianship, I draw inspiration from the legacy left by our elders in the field. Among these pioneers, Edward C. Williams (1871-1929) stands as America's first Black librarian, advocating tirelessly to address challenges faced by Black libraries historically. While serving as the head librarian at Howard University, he pursued a doctorate at Columbia University, a pursuit he didn't get to celebrate due to his untimely death. Clara Stanton Jones (1913-2012), the first Black president of the American Library Association, dedicated her life to desegregating libraries and promoting awareness of racism and sexism within the profession. Dorothy B. Porter (1905-1995), the first Black American graduate of Columbia University's Library School in 1932, challenged the Dewey Decimal System with her innovative classification method, unveiling inherent racism within library science. And this is just to name a few. Their collective contributions underscore the power of the ways literature has uplifted, empowered, and united communities.

In Shirley A. Wiegand and Wayne A. Wiegand's *The Desegregation of Public Libraries in the Jim Crow South: Civil Rights and Local Activism*, readers are reminded of the advocacy it took to ensure the Black community had access to books. One quote from the text resonates deeply with me:

> Librarian Annie Watters McPheeters, who had been refused library service as a child, later recalled: "I have fond memories of those [book mobile] stations, one in particular. It was under a large spreading oak tree near a country church. . . . I could see [people] coming down the road and across the field. The books they were returning were carefully wrapped in newspaper or in a brown paper bag for protection while they worked in the field or elsewhere. To watch them as they left with their selections from the bookmobile gave me an inner joy hard to explain."

The "library as community place" model established by Louisville's Thomas Fountain Blue (1866-1935) became a blueprint for Black librarians who sought to establish community centers, providing a range of different services at the local library. During what was named the Black "public library movement" in Alabama in the 1940s and 1950s, local community leaders, educators, Black civic organizations, and churches all collaborated to make quality literature accessible and to provide free services to the community via the public library. Black library branches provided books to local classrooms at Black schools because of segregation laws that would not allow the main branches to provide bookmobile services to Black folks.

Libraries have always been pillars of both individual and community mental health. They were then and they are now. In addition, libraries are the lifeblood of our communities, offering an array of vital services that extend far beyond book lending. In marginalized communities, often referred to as literary deserts, where local bookstores are scarce or nonexistent (such as in the Bronx), libraries play an irreplaceable role. They serve as knowledge hubs, providing access to books, educational resources, and digital technology; they narrow the digital divide and bolster digital literacy.

Libraries offer a platform for community organizing, fostering public health by hosting workshops, events, and resources related to physical and mental well-being. From literacy programs for children to job-search assistance for adults, libraries offer tools for upward mobility, empowering individuals to improve their quality of life. In the tapestry of marginalized communities, libraries are not just institutions; they are essential community anchors that facilitate learning, connection, and access to information—a ray of optimism in the midst of literary deserts.

The desegregation of libraries provided platforms for Black authors, poets, and intellectuals to share their work, and gave Black readers access to a wider range of literature that reflected our identities, histories, and perspectives as part of the larger Civil Rights Movement that sought to challenge and dismantle racial segregation and discrimination. We have a long way to go, and thanks to pioneers such as those mentioned above, we have a roadmap.

EMPOWERING AFRICAN AMERICAN YOUTH THROUGH CULTURALLY AFFIRMING BIBLIOTHERAPY

Highlighting the crucial role of Black librarians in addressing the impact of race on children and adolescents of African descent underscores the necessity of diverse representation in library spaces. Race profoundly affects every aspect of the lives of individuals of African descent, shaping our perceptions of ourselves and our interactions with society.

Pervasive societal standards, often rooted in middle-class and European American norms, frequently result in African American youth feeling marginalized or inadequately represented. These challenges are compounded by racial stereotypes perpetuated by the media, which often depict African American males as criminals and females as overly sexualized. These harmful portrayals, deeply ingrained in our social consciousness, contribute to the internalization of negative stereotypes and the erosion of self-esteem among African American youth.

Culturally affirming bibliotherapy, facilitated by Black librarians, serves as a vital tool in combating these damaging narratives and promoting positive racial identity development. By providing access to literature that reflects and affirms their experiences, Black librarians empower African American youth to navigate and challenge societal expectations, fostering resilience and self-determination in the face of adversity. Recognizing the significance of representation and culturally relevant resources in library spaces underscores the critical role of Black librarians in supporting the mental health and well-being of African American communities.

Young adult librarians, in particular, play a unique and vital role in cultivating reading experiences that resonate with adolescents navigating the complexities of youth. They serve as guides and mentors, curating book collections that reflect diverse perspectives and address the multifaceted interests and concerns of young readers. When selecting and recommending books, these librarians consider literary merit as well as relevance to the lived experiences of their audience. They actively seek out titles that feature diverse characters, cultures, and backgrounds, recognizing the significance of representation in fostering empathy, understanding, and a sense of belonging. Through their recommendations, young adult librarians aim to empower readers to explore new worlds, perspectives, and ideas, fostering a lifelong love of reading and learning.

Young adult programming is another cornerstone of the librarian's role, providing opportunities for teens to engage with literature, culture, and community in dynamic and meaningful ways. From book clubs and author visits to creative writing workshops and cultural events, these programs offer spaces for young people to connect, share, and explore their identities and interests. Librarians collaborate with educators, community leaders, and youth advocates to design programming that is inclusive, relevant, and accessible to all. By fostering a sense of belonging and empowerment, young adult librarians help teens develop critical-thinking skills, build social connections, and discover their voices in an ever-changing world.

DIVERSE VOICES IN YOUNG ADULT LITERATURE

Title: The Crossover by Kwame Alexander
Why Librarians Recommend It:

The Crossover is an innovative novel-in-verse that resonates with readers of all ages, particularly young people navigating the complexities of adolescence. Written by celebrated author Kwame Alexander, this Newbery Medal–winning book tells the story of twin brothers Josh and Jordan Bell, talented basketball players who must navigate family dynamics, friendship, and the challenges of growing up.

Librarians recommend *The Crossover* for its captivating narrative style, which combines poetry, rhythm, and sports to create a unique reading experience. Through the lens of basketball, Alexander addresses universal themes such as sibling rivalry, identity, and the bonds of family, making the story relatable and engaging for readers from diverse backgrounds.

As Josh grapples with the pressures of competition, love, and loss, readers are drawn into his world, experiencing the highs and lows of his journey both on and off the court. *The Crossover* celebrates the power of poetry and storytelling to capture the rhythm and energy of life while also addressing important issues such as friendship, grief, and resilience.

Librarians recognize *The Crossover* as an essential addition to any young-adult collection, particularly for Black youth seeking literature that reflects their experiences and celebrates the beauty of Black culture. By providing access to diverse and inclusive stories like *The Crossover*, librarians empower African American youth to see themselves represented in literature and find inspiration in the power of storytelling.

Title: *Ghost* by Jason Reynolds
Why Librarians Recommend It:

Ghost is the first installment in Jason Reynolds' acclaimed Track series, which follows a group of young athletes as they navigate the challenges of life and sports. In this novel, Reynolds introduces readers to Castle "Ghost" Cranshaw, a troubled youth with a gift for running who finds redemption on the track.

Librarians recommend *Ghost* for its authentic portrayal of the struggles and triumphs faced by young people growing up in urban communities. Through Castle's journey, Reynolds addresses themes of identity, resilience, and the power of mentorship, offering readers a relatable and inspiring story of transformation.

As Castle grapples with past traumas and strives to overcome obstacles both on and off the track, readers are drawn into his world, rooting for his success and growth. Reynolds' dynamic storytelling and engaging characters make *Ghost* a compelling read for readers of all ages, encouraging empathy, reflection, and dialogue.

Librarians recognize that *Ghost* is especially powerful for Black youth seeking stories that reflect their experiences, as it celebrates the strength and resilience of Black communities. By providing access to diverse and empowering narratives like *Ghost*, librarians empower African American youth to see themselves reflected in literature and find inspiration in stories of perseverance and hope.

Title: *Brown Girl Dreaming* by Jacqueline Woodson
Why Librarians Recommend It:

This memoir-in-verse follows the author's childhood experiences growing up as an African American girl in the 1960s and 1970s. Through poetry, Woodson explores themes of family, identity, and the Civil Rights Movement, offering a relatable and empowering narrative for young Black readers to connect with their heritage and embrace their stories.

The book also aligns with the four main goals of bibliotherapy in clinical practice. First, *Brown Girl Dreaming* facilitates increased self-understanding by providing representation and validation for young readers. Woodson's reflection on her childhood experiences speaks to the significance of seeing oneself reflected in literature. As the protagonist shares, "If someone had taken / that book out of my hand / said, you're too old for this / maybe / I'd never have believed / that someone who looked like me / could be in the pages of the book / that someone who looked like me / had a story."

Brown Girl Dreaming contributes to improving reality orientation by grounding readers in the vivid landscapes of memory and imagination. Through Woodson's lyrical prose, readers are transported to the South, where the sun always shines in Daddy's garden, providing a sense of nostalgia and connection to place.

This book enriches internal images and enhances the capacity to respond by encouraging readers to listen to the stories within silence. Woodson's evocative language prompts readers to tune into the subtle narratives embedded in everyday moments. As she writes, "Even the silence / has a story to tell you. / Just listen. Listen."

Brown Girl Dreaming increases awareness of interpersonal relationships by exploring themes of race, identity, and belonging. Through vivid vignettes, Woodson explores the complexities of navigating a racially segregated society, offering insights into the challenges faced by African American families. As the protagonist grapples with societal expectations and racial injustice, readers are encouraged to reflect on their own relationships and identities. As Woodson writes, "Even though the laws have changed / my grandmother still takes us / to the back of the bus when we go downtown / in the rain . . . I look around and see the ones / who walk straight to the back . . . And know / this is who I want to be. Not scared / like that. Brave / like that."

Brown Girl Dreaming serves as a powerful tool for cultural affirmation and healing. Through its exploration of self, reality, response, and relationships, Woodson's memoir invites readers on a journey of introspection and empathy that helps them cultivate a connection to intergenerational healing and a deeper understanding of self and others.

ANDREW CARNEGIE

As we reflect on the exploration of culturally affirming titles, which are intentionally chosen by librarians who curate a reading space that feels like home to a library's constituents, it's essential to understand the profound impact of literature and libraries on communities. One individual whose philanthropic efforts have significantly shaped the landscape of public libraries is Andrew Carnegie.

Born in Scotland in 1835, Carnegie immigrated with his family to the United States, where he would become one of the wealthiest industrialists of his time. However, Carnegie's legacy extends far beyond his business success. Inspired by his humble beginnings and a belief in the power of education, he dedicated a substantial portion of his wealth to establishing public libraries across the United States and beyond. His vision was to make knowledge and literature accessible, thus democratizing learning and honing community development.

Through his philanthropic leadership, Andrew Carnegie played a significant role in making libraries accessible to the public. Here are some ways in which Carnegie's contributions to library development—commonly known as the Carnegie library movement—contributed to making libraries accessible to the public:

- *Funding Library Buildings*: Carnegie believed libraries should be public institutions that provide free access to books and educational resources. Between 1883 and 1929, his philanthropic endeavors resulted in the establishment of more than 2,500 Carnegie libraries, including the construction of the buildings and the initial book collections.
- *Cooperative Approach*: Carnegie required local communities to demonstrate their commitment to providing ongoing financial support for library operations and maintenance. Communities were expected to allocate funds for staff salaries, book acquisitions, and general upkeep.

- *Accessibility and Inclusivity*: Carnegie emphasized the importance of making libraries accessible to all members of the community, regardless of their social or economic status. His libraries were open to the public, free of charge, and often situated in central locations to ensure ease of access. This made libraries available to people who might not otherwise have had access to books or educational resources.
- *Standardized Design*: Carnegie libraries often followed a standardized design plan, known as the Carnegie library architectural style. This design made the buildings recognizable and efficient, featuring specific architectural elements and layout considerations that aimed to maximize functionality and usability.
- *Educational Programming*: While Carnegie primarily focused on providing library infrastructure, many of the libraries built with his funding also offered educational programming and resources. These included lectures, community events, and opportunities for self-improvement.

Carnegie's contributions significantly expanded public access to books and educational resources, making libraries more accessible and available to communities. Through his philanthropy, Carnegie had a lasting impact on public library systems, contributing to the growth and development of public libraries as vital community institutions—repositories for books as well as centers of cultural enrichment, lifelong learning, and social connection. Today, Carnegie's legacy continues to resonate, reminding us of the enduring importance of libraries as pillars of knowledge, inclusion, and empowerment in our communities.

I often tell my clients that when friends and family judge them for adding to a never-ending to-be-read book stack, they could remind the critics that, not so long ago, it was only a privilege of the elite to have a personal library. While philanthropists like Carnegie helped to make libraries accessible to the public, Carnegie didn't always support labor unions. While he did fund a lot of libraries, these libraries weren't always accessible to everyone, sometimes excluding certain racial or ethnic groups. It's important to see both the good and not-so-good aspects of Carnegie's philanthropy and how it impacted society. It's also important to honor that, as we build our personal libraries, we are engaging in an act of reclamation and access to ease and knowledge that our ancestors did not have. And it's important that we make the connection that when we buy or borrow books, we are providing ourselves with opportunities for growth and healing that our ancestors did not have.

BIBLIOTHERAPEUTIC REFLECTION:

1. Reflect on your personal experiences with the public library. How has the library served as a bridge to well-being in your life? Consider the books, programs, or resources that have had a significant effect on your overall well-being.

2. In what ways can you contribute to the vitality of your local library? Reflect on specific actions you can take to support and enhance the library's role as a community hub for well-being. This may include participating in library programs, signing up your students or loved ones for a library card, advocating for increased funding, or volunteering your time and skills.

3. How can you share the benefits of the library with others in your community? Consider creative ways to spread awareness about the positive impact of libraries on well-being, and encourage others to explore the diverse resources and services available. Reflect on the potential ripple effects your advocacy could have on community members' overall sense of fulfillment and connection.

CHAPTER 3

WORDS AS WITNESSES

I hear hints of Grandpa's wisdom; I hear words like rest, heal, with whispers of repeated patience.

—ARI TISON, *Saints of the Household*

As Daniel Black astutely notes, "In the midst of trauma, remembering is difficult." This statement speaks to the profound emotional challenge we face when navigating traumatic memories. Within this struggle to recollect, confront, and comprehend, the significance of words as witnesses becomes abundantly clear.

Language, with its transfiguring capabilities, offers us a tool for meaning-making and understanding in the aftermath of traumatic events. Words become the vessel through which we navigate the tumultuous seas of our experiences. In the face of adversity, words help us bear witness to our own stories and connect us to the narratives of others who have walked similar paths. This interconnectedness through language fosters a collective strength, allowing individuals to share, understand, and heal in unison. As we explore the profound role of words as witnesses, we illuminate the pathways through which language becomes a guiding force in the journey toward recovery.

As we explored in the last chapter, beyond its contemporary manifestation within civil rights advocacy, the roots of bibliotherapy—especially with respect to revealing the power of our language to shape
our reality and help us bear witness to our complex histories—can
be found in traditions of librarianship. As we further consider the
profound impact of bibliotherapy on our emotional well-being, this
next chapter will closely examine the healing mechanism of literature. In this exploration, I introduce Arleen McCarty Hynes (1916–
2006), a distinguished librarian and pioneering bibliotherapist
whose pivotal role in shaping the field is underscored by her establishment of the inaugural training program for bibliotherapy in hospital settings in 1974. We also delve into the four key goals I shared
earlier, which were formulated by Hynes and serve as guiding principles in the practical application of bibliotherapy in clinical
contexts.

ARLEEN MCCARTY HYNES

Hynes was among the first to develop the programmatic aspect of
books for healing in general hospitals, where patients would have
access to a library to peruse for their reading pleasure. Through her
work, she helped hospitals recognize the value of bibliotherapy in
improving patients' mental health in a medical setting. Hynes differ-
entiated prescribing books for treatment (prescriptive bibliotherapy)
from reading books together during sessions in treatment (interactive bibliotherapy). Her book *Biblio/Poetry Therapy: The Interactive
Process: A Handbook* is a classic text for those studying the core
method of bibliotherapy.

The four main goals of bibliotherapy that I refer to in Chapter 1
are outlined in Hynes' book and frame the science behind understanding how books help us heal. In her article "The Arts in
Psychotherapy" (1980), she writes about how literature provides
readers with ways of coping more gracefully and ideas for generating
creative solutions to life's problems.

In other words, when we read, we are doing so much more than escaping our daily realities to enjoy the pleasures of being transported to another place and time. We are healing ourselves. We are learning to be more mindful and to savor the present moment. We are sitting with our feelings and reflecting on our relationships. We are improving our ability to understand what we think and how we authentically feel so that we can better respond to the world and the people around us. Books help connect us to self, and therefore, books help connect us to each other.

Hynes also established the four steps of the bibliotherapeutic process for clinical work and became the first president of the National Federation for Biblio/Poetry Therapy (NFB/PT), an organization she helped develop to set the standards in the field of bibliotherapy and poetry therapy. Hynes wrote that the four-step process for an individual to be helped using literature is as follows:

1. *Recognition*: The client must connect with some aspect of the literature.
2. *Examination*: The client considers the personal feeling response they are having because of the themes and issues presented in the text.
3. *Juxtaposition*: The client moves to the next level of understanding the connections they've made between their personal experiences and the text. Through engaging in a discussion facilitated by the therapist, the client brings their awareness to any unexpected feelings or ideas that are emerging.
4. *Self-Application*: The client analyzes and evaluates the impressions and new insights they've gained from reading with the therapist and integrates this new knowledge into their inner self (thoughts, feelings, wants, needs, etc.).

The objective of clinical bibliotherapy is always to help bottled-up emotions not in our conscious awareness rise to the surface. It is less about the cognitive act of intellectualizing and more about the intentional act of allowing a feeling response to happen. Once emotions arise, we can become curious about what that feeling response might teach us about who we are, what we feel, and what we need.

Incorporating literature into therapy proves highly effective in facilitating clients' emotional expression. It encourages them to directly acknowledge, label, and convey their feelings. These expressions can take various forms, from moments of profound silence to tears and, at times, even outbursts of screaming or shouting. I've been there to offer support when clients needed to curl up in the fetal position, providing a comforting presence during their most vulnerable moments. In a society that often encourages emotional detachment in the pursuit of productivity and capitalism, our capacity for emotional well-being and intelligence is frequently underdeveloped, if not outright resisted. Sometimes, the words can show us the way to honor our innermost emotions. Sometimes, the words can be witnesses.

Among Hynes' significant contributions to the field of bibliotherapy, she established the first training program for bibliotherapy in hospital settings. The guidelines and protocols she developed for implementing bibliotherapy programs in hospital settings addressed issues such as book selection, creating reading spaces, and training health care professionals in the practice of bibliotherapy. She focused on integrating bibliotherapy into health care environments to support patients' emotional well-being. Hynes also emphasized the importance of collaboration between librarians, health care providers, and mental health professionals to implement effective bibliotherapy programs. Her groundbreaking work at St. Elizabeth's Hospital in Washington, D.C. did much to legitimize the modality of using books to heal.

CLINICAL BIBLIOTHERAPY: THE CASE OF EVELYN | *HALSEY STREET* BY NAIMA COSTER

During a bibliotherapy session I curated for a client, Evelyn, who was working on healing her mother wound, I pulled from the book *Halsey Street* by Naima Coster. The mother wound, as viewed by mental health professionals, refers to the emotional and psychological impact of unresolved issues or traumas stemming from the mother/child relationship, which can include feelings of abandonment, neglect, or unmet needs that influence an individual's emotional well-being and interpersonal relationships. Addressing and understanding these early childhood dynamics can be crucial in the therapeutic process to promote healing and personal growth. Evelyn is a voracious reader, and incorporating literature into our work together proved to be an effective intervention because of the previous difficulty she had verbalizing her emotional challenges.

Halsey Street is a novel that delves deep into the complexities of family, identity, and the intricacies of mother/daughter relationships. The story revolves around Penelope Grand, a talented artist living in Pittsburgh, who returns to her childhood home in the Brooklyn neighborhood of Bedford-Stuyvesant. The decision to return is driven by a desire to care for her ailing father, but it also opens old wounds and reveals the fractured bond between Penelope and her mother, Mirella.

Mother/daughter estrangement is a central theme of the novel, stemming from a tumultuous history of misunderstandings, missed opportunities for communication, and unspoken resentments. Mirella's aspirations for Penelope clash with her daughter's desire for independence and creative freedom, leading to a painful rift. As Penelope grapples with her artistic ambitions and confronts the challenges of gentrification reshaping her childhood neighborhood, her strained relationship with her mother is a constant, haunting presence in her life.

Coster masterfully portrays this estrangement, weaving it into the fabric of the story to explore themes of heritage, gentrification, and the struggle for self-identity. *Halsey Street* is a poignant and beauti-fully written narrative that explores the emotional complexities of family ties. It offers a nuanced portrayal of the enduring love and tension between a mother and daughter as they navigate their shared history and uncertain future.

The quote I pulled for my bibliotherapy session with Evelyn was this one:

> Penelope thought of her grandmother and drank again from the flask. She closed her eyes and conjured up the old woman, held her close. She was dead and yet she was nearer to Penelope than Mirella had ever been. She couldn't say whether she had once loved her mother, only that she had once pined for her mother's love. She reminded herself that she had not come to pine again—she would get what she came for and then leave. It was simple. It was easy.

I asked Evelyn if she'd like to read the book's quote aloud or if she'd like me to. I always ask this question to respect the way the client prefers to engage with the text and with me. She asked if she could read it, but in silence to herself. When she finished reading, she au-dibly sighed. I remained quiet, holding the space. I waited for what felt like five minutes or so, aware that if I spoke first, it would derail the acknowledgment of whatever Evelyn was feeling.

"I know that feeling" were the first words out of her mouth in response to the text.

"Which one?" I asked.

"The feeling of pining for my mother's love," she responded tearfully.

"Can you describe it for me?" I asked gently.

"It's like being dehydrated and your mother being the only one who could get you a glass of water. It's like she's taunting me by hold-ing the water in her hand and ignoring that my arms are outstretched, reaching for a sip," she explained.

"Would your grandmother have given you the water?" I asked.

"My grandmother would have anticipated I was thirsty before she would have ever allowed me to become dehydrated," she said.

For the remainder of our session together, we processed how much her grandmother's love differed from her mother's. I spoke very little, only responding by asking questions to help Evelyn draw deeper connections between her life and the text. She spoke to me about the intimacy she felt with her grandmother and how cold her mother could be to her, even as a little girl. She made the connection between the rejection she felt and how her drinking habit formed as a coping mechanism to numb painful memories when they surfaced. Most importantly, she allowed herself to be seen and held by me. Reading Mirella and Penelope's story helped her sit with her truth and share it vulnerably with me in a way that felt safer than it would have without a fictional reference point.

BIBLIOTHERAPY
THE PROCESS

1. Engaging with the text.

2. Identification with a character.

3. Emotional catharsis.

4. Adult-led discussion and insights gained.

5. Universalization of insights gained.

UNLOCKING EMOTIONAL NARRATIVES:
THE TRANSFORMATIVE JOURNEY OF BIBLIOTHERAPY

In my sessions with Evelyn, an avid reader grappling with the complexities of her family dynamics, we looked at the profound impact of her grandmother's love compared to the coldness she experienced from her mother. Encouraging her to understand these emotions, I chose a minimalist approach, using carefully selected questions to guide Evelyn in drawing connections from the text she immersed herself in. Through Mirella and Penelope's story, Evelyn found safe passage to articulate her own truth, allowing vulnerability to take root in our therapeutic space.

In facilitating Evelyn's bibliotherapy session focused on healing her mother wound, the narrative, which centers around Penelope's complex relationship with her mother, Mirella, provided a mirror for Evelyn to connect with her own experiences of maternal estrangement. As Evelyn silently absorbed heartfelt quotes from the novel, her most authentic emotions about her experiences were allowed to rise to the surface in the safety of the therapy room. When Evelyn was invited to articulate her reaction, she expressed a profound recognition of her longing for maternal love, comparing it to the metaphor of being dehydrated, with her mother holding the water just out of reach. This revelation enabled Evelyn to draw insightful connections between her grandmother's nurturing love and her mother's emotional distance.

Throughout the session, the fictional enabled Evelyn to vulnerably access and share her truth. By guiding her to explore these insights, we collectively navigated the healing journey—from connecting with a character's experience, facilitating emotional catharsis, and drawing meaningful insights to ultimately incorporating newfound understanding into Evelyn's daily life and mindset. The power of bibliotherapy was evident. Evelyn felt seen, allowing her to confront and process her narrative with a depth of understanding and self-awareness that transcended the boundaries of fiction.

Engaging with literature offers a unique pathway to access our unconscious thoughts, feelings, and fears. As readers immerse themselves in a story, they form emotional connections with characters and themes, naturally fostering empathy and introspection without self-judgment. Evelyn's experience underscores the potency of storytelling, revealing how literature acts as a bridge to universal experiences and emotions that resonate with our shadow aspects.

ARCHETYPES:
MIRRORS TO THE SOUL

Within the pages of literature, archetypes serve as universal symbols, reflecting fundamental human experiences and emotions. Rooted in Jungian psychology, archetypes provide a framework for understanding the collective unconscious—a concept explored by Carl Jung. Recognizing and understanding these archetypes allows readers to consciously connect with the emotions stirred by their lived experiences. For instance, the "Hero" archetype may evoke admiration and inspiration, mirroring a reader's journey of overcoming obstacles. In contrast, the "Trickster" archetype might prompt amusement or discomfort, resonating with those who have encountered cunning individuals in their lives. Readers like Evelyn experience emotional catharsis, release, understanding, and validation for their own inner struggles when they engage with texts that are rich with archetypes.

Clarissa Pinkola Estés, a Jungian psychologist and author of *Women Who Run with the Wolves*, deepens our understanding of archetypes. In her work, she emphasizes the retrieval of intuition as an initiation into right relationship with our self and our truest desires. By reconnecting to the wild woman (being) within, Estés urges us to look inside ourselves to obtain clarity about our longings. She shares archetypal symbols, myths, fables, and allegorical stories from different cultures to encourage readers to reclaim what has been lost of our true nature due to the impact of colonialism and systems of oppression (such as capitalism or the carceral state) that keep us in constant motion and reinforce depersonalization.

Estés captures the essence of what bibliotherapy means to me in one statement: "In all tales, there is material that can be understood as a mirror reflecting the illnesses or the well-being of one's culture or one's own inner life."

Through the symbolic language of archetypes in literature, readers like Evelyn confront their deepest emotions and engage in a process of cultural and personal introspection, leading to a richer understanding of themselves and their place in the world. Bibliotherapy, as a result, becomes a profound tool for self-reflection and healing (or gathering the bones, in Estés' words), guided by the wisdom embedded in the pages we read.

Fairy tales especially hold strong archetypal themes, mirroring the timeless struggles and triumphs inherent in the human experience. The choice to incorporate the fairy tale "Hansel and Gretel" into my work with Evelyn was deliberate, as this narrative contained relevant archetypes and tropes, such as the Hero (whose saga is often referred to as the "Hero's Journey"), the Shadow, and the Sibling Bond. By immersing Evelyn in the symbolic landscape of "Hansel and Gretel," which we'll explore in the next section, she found a resonant mirror for her own grief over losing her brother, Gabriel, who served as her hero. Through the shared emotional terrain of the fairy tale, Evelyn and I journeyed on a cathartic exploration, allowing her to process and integrate the complexities of her loss within the framework of a universally understood narrative.

Evelyn's journey exemplifies how bibliotherapy provides a secure and reflective space for individuals to explore their unconscious without the fear of judgment. This therapeutic approach becomes a supportive tool, both clinically, for addressing emotional challenges, and developmentally, for identifying areas of growth and acquiring new skills. Through the alchemy of literature, readers like Evelyn confront their deepest emotions and embark on a revelatory journey of increased self-compassion and understanding.

DEVELOPMENTAL BIBLIOTHERAPY:
EVELYN'S CHILDHOOD | "HANSEL AND GRETEL"

When I first met Evelyn, one of the first things she mentioned on her reading intake was that her favorite childhood story was "Hansel and Gretel." I immediately wondered about her sibling relationships and the dynamics therein. "Hansel and Gretel" is a classic fairy tale about the two titular siblings and their harrowing encounter with a wicked witch in the woods. The tale begins with a poor woodcutter and his wife who decide to abandon their children in the forest due to a severe famine. The parents, struggling to feed their family, reluctantly leave the two children behind, thinking they will have a better chance of survival on their own. Super shady, I know! But this was also relevant to the theme of parental rejection that Evelyn had processed in a previous session, so I knew that incorporating this fairy tale into our work together would be meaningful.

The sibling dynamic between Hansel and Gretel is one of profound loyalty and mutual support. It was the same strong bond, I soon learned, that Evelyn shared growing up with her brother before he passed away in a car accident at the age of twenty-two. Hansel and Gretel hold onto each other tightly in their moment of abandonment, their bond unbreakable. Evelyn and her brother, Gabriel, looked out for each other even when their mother neglected their needs for connection and play.

It took more than a year of therapy sessions with Evelyn before she broached the topic of her brother's tragic passing. The catalyst for this conversation was a chance encounter during a Target shopping trip. In the children's book section, she stumbled upon a volume of fairy tales that triggered a flood of memories. As she gazed at the cover, the image of a witch invoked recollections of the childhood games she and Gabriel used to play. In these imaginative scenarios, Gabriel would take on the role of her hero, rescuing her from the clutches of the wicked witch. Evelyn, in turn, would assume the role of the damsel in distress, pretending to be trapped in her closet as her brother masterfully wove an impromptu narrative that unfailingly concluded with her rescue.

Gabriel's portrayal as the hero in these make-believe adventures resonated deeply with Evelyn. It was during this phase of her therapeutic journey that she explored and processed the impact of her brother's untimely departure. The enduring emotional charge of the Hero archetype, intertwined with the fairy tale of "Hansel and

Gretel," continues to summon powerful emotions within Evelyn, serving as a testament to the enduring influence of the stories and relationships that shape our lives.

In the fairy tale, Hansel, the older brother, assumes a protective role, leaving a trail of breadcrumbs to guide their way home. However, this plan fails when the breadcrumbs are eaten by birds, leaving Hansel and Gretel lost in the woods. As they venture deeper into the forest, Hansel and Gretel stumble upon a gingerbread house inhabited by a seemingly kind old woman. Unbeknownst to them, the woman is a witch who intends to capture and eat them. Hansel and Gretel use their wits and courage to outsmart the witch and find their way back home. Similarly, Evelyn and Gabriel engaged in pretend play to infuse joy into a home life that was otherwise cold and disconnected.

The tale of "Hansel and Gretel" underscores the enduring strength of the sibling bond, as the two children rely on each other to overcome adversity and escape the clutches of the malevolent witch. It is a story of resilience, resourcefulness, and the unwavering love between brother and sister in the face of grave danger—and, one might say, in the absence of social support for vulnerable children, which is a stark reality that persists to this day. The story allowed Evelyn to introduce me to the memory of her brother in a way that allowed her defenses to lower and her grief to have a voice in the therapy room.

INNER-CHILD HEALING AND CHILDREN'S LITERATURE

In my experience, I have learned that inner-child healing is supported by the use of children's books when working with adult clients. Fairy tales, originally containing adult themes, harbor darker realities beneath their surface. This makes these allegorical tales powerful bibliotherapy selections across the lifespan. "Hansel and Gretel," a classic Grimm Brothers' tale, is a narrative laden with adult content such as climate change, famine, and survival cannibalism. Its medieval German setting reflects the harsh realities of historical famines, emphasizing the desperate measures families had to take to survive.

The evolving versions of the story, culminating in the 1857 edition, maintain the core thread of familial betrayal and hardship. Despite their simplicity, children's books possess a profound capacity to resonate with the nuances of adult experiences. Revisiting these tales allows adults to access a symbolic realm that transcends age, offering a bridge to childhood memories, emotions, and imagination. In this way, fairy tales become a therapeutic tool, guiding adult clients toward reconnection with their childhood selves.

In a sense, incorporating the use of books that adults enjoyed as children allows the inner child to take center stage. A twinkle appears in the eye of every adult I've counseled using children's literature. Maybe it's the agency they feel in making the story their own again—except this time, as it relates to the meaning of adulting, as well as the desire for a reconnection to play and adventure. Maybe it's that the books we read as children remind us of a less complicated time when we may have been nurtured and allowed to engage our creativity without the judgment of a world that only places value on how much we produce. Either way, reading children's books as a form of developmental bibliotherapy is an effective intervention to bring a client's inner child into the room.

Exploring a client's inner child through the lens of childhood stories serves a therapeutic purpose. It aligns with the broader understanding that gaining insight into the inner child illuminates unmet needs and experiences from our childhoods. When we are children, we have a psychic need to idealize our parents and caregivers, and we overlook their faults and imperfections to maintain a sense of safety within. As adults, we can look at the past with more objectivity and clearly see what we needed that we didn't get—not in a way that judges our parents but in a way that helps us better understand the truth of the matter.

As clients engage in bibliotherapy, revisiting tales like "Hansel and Gretel" becomes a vehicle for reflection on their childhood memories. The narrative elements resonate with the complexities of the past and allow feelings about the past to rise to the surface. Making connections between the past and the present helps us understand why we behave the way we do and where our core beliefs come from. These connections provide more clarity about what sorts of changes we hope to make and how to go about making them as adults now fully in control of our lives.

DEVELOPMENTAL BIBLIOTHERAPY

Developmental bibliotherapy (which we've explored throughout this book so far) is a term coined by Glenn H. Darrow, a psychologist and educator who popularized the concept in the 1950s and 1960s. He emphasized the use of carefully selected books to promote emotional and intellectual growth in children and adolescents. Darrow's work focused on utilizing literature as a tool for personal development, self-reflection, and emotional education, particularly during the formative stages of childhood and adolescence. His contributions laid the foundation for the practice of developmental bibliotherapy and its integration into educational and counseling settings.

Many teachers have not considered that the work they are doing while teaching literature is bibliotherapeutic. Any caring educator who teaches beyond the curriculum to help students make meaning out of their experiences is helping their students heal and teaching them new skills. The emotionally responsive classroom is the most accessible community of all, and we learn and heal best in community. In the words of ancestor bell hooks, "Rarely, if ever, are any of us healed in isolation. Healing is an act of communion."

When we acknowledge that all children are mandated to attend school, it becomes clear that the classroom serves as a pivotal arena where educators can enact meaningful interventions for all students. By consciously crafting a classroom atmosphere characterized by emotional responsiveness, warmth, and developmental appropriateness, we establish an ideal environment for healing.

In a developmentally appropriate and emotionally responsive classroom, children acquire knowledge and partake in a collective process. This communal space offers them the social and emotional support essential for their growth into the individuals they are destined to become—a vital complement to the support they may or may not receive at home. Like my first-grade teacher, Ms. Parkins, the teachers we meet in childhood who are key figures along the course of our development become part of our internalized representations of interpersonal relationships. We start to develop a worldview inclusive of the goodness that exists in others, despite what we may not have received from our families of origin.

BIBLIOTHERAPY IN THE CLASSROOM ENVIRONMENT

James Forgan is an educator who developed a helpful framework for understanding how to engage students when reading a text and experiencing their own form of emotional connection and catharsis. A child's capacity to experience emotional connection forms the foundation for lifelong well-being, as these early connections shape our understanding of self and others. Healthy emotional bonds established in childhood foster a sense of security, resilience, and the ability to navigate relationships with trust and empathy. This contributes to positive mental and emotional development. The emotional connections formed in our early years serve as a blueprint for later relationships, influencing our capacity for intimacy, communication, and overall mental health throughout our lives.

There are four main steps to incorporating bibliotherapy in the classroom. In the prereading stage, teachers choose a text relevant to their students' experience. Teachers provide background knowledge of the story and context while asking students to make predictions about what they anticipate will happen in the story. This prompts reflection and gets students to start thinking about connections between the story and their own lives.

Moving into the second phase, guided reading, the teacher reads the story aloud, and the students listen attentively. In the third phase, post-reading, teachers assess for comprehension and engage students in a discussion about the story's problems and solutions. In the final stage, problem-solving, students identify solutions and barriers in the story and reflect on their own preferred solutions. This is a great time to ask students if they see any similarities between how characters respond to their challenges and how they themselves would react. If applying the situation to their lives feels challenging, creating role-play situations is a powerful activity to get students to learn new skills and apply valuable lessons to their lives and what the book is teaching.

But the real magic happens in the post-reading discussion, the third step of Forgan's framework. Here, teachers can check for comprehension, delve into the story's problems and solutions, and guide students through the process of identification, catharsis, and resolution. By facilitating these discussions, teachers create a space for students to share their thoughts, feelings, and experiences, ultimately supporting their emotional growth and well-being. The process teaches language and literacy as well as empathy, resilience, and self-awareness, equipping students with essential life skills and fostering a deeper understanding of themselves and the world around them.

FINDING MY VOICE: MAYA ANGELOU'S TRANSFORMATIVE INFLUENCE ON MY JOURNEY THROUGH GIRLHOOD

It was my eighth-grade teacher who introduced me to Maya Angelou. I found *I Know Why the Caged Bird Sings* in my English Language Arts classroom. It was an introduction to an author whose work would prove life-changing and healing for me in many ways as I grew up in a tumultuous environment marked by domestic violence, unaddressed mental health issues, and my personal encounters with colorism, racism, and discrimination. This book played a vital role in shedding light on the strength of the human spirit—topics rarely broached by the adults in my life. Through Angelou's story, I discovered affirmation for the emotions and questions swirling within me.

One particular revelation that left a profound mark was Angelou's exploration of the values held dear within the Black community, as well as our practice of employing different languages in various contexts. For the first time, I grasped the concept of code-switching as a survival skill acquired by those of us navigating life within racialized bodies. This newfound understanding expanded my worldview and provided a lens through which to comprehend the complexities of the world around me. Angelou's literary masterpiece became a catalyst for healing, guiding me on a journey of self-understanding and empowerment that would resonate throughout my life.

She writes:

> My education and that of my Black associates were quite different from the education of our white schoolmates. In the classroom we all learned past participles, but in the streets and in our homes the Blacks learned to drop the s's from plurals and suffixes from past tense verbs. . . . At school, in a given situation, we might respond with "That's not unusual." But in the street, meeting the same situation, we easily said, "It be's like that sometimes."

Reading *I Know Why the Caged Bird Sings* provided comforting validation and a valuable lesson in the power of literature to illuminate the truths that society sometimes chooses to keep hidden. I learned that the way I spoke wasn't wrong. I just needed to learn to speak multiple languages. *I Know Why the Caged Bird Sings* became more than just a book; it was a guiding light on my journey to understanding the world, my place in it, and the importance of embracing my own Black body, language, and identity. This book also prepared me to be a witness to my clients' stories and understand their unique ways of navigating their worlds through language.

BIBLIOTHERAPY IN PRISONS

Bibliotherapy helps individuals in many ways by providing a North Star in dark places. The use of books to heal within the confines of prison is also a powerful testament to the transformative potential of reading literature. A striking example of this healing power can be found in the life story of author Shaka Senghor. While serving time, including periods in solitary confinement, Senghor discovered healing and redemption through reading and writing.

His journey from incarceration to becoming an acclaimed author of two books, including *Writing My Wrongs: Life, Death, and Redemption in an American Prison*, exemplifies the profound impact books can have on individuals seeking personal growth and rehabilitation. Senghor's narrative underscores the cathartic nature of reading and writing and highlights its ability to cultivate empathy, self-reflection, and healing, even in the most challenging and dehumanizing circumstances. His story serves as a potent reminder that the written word can be a lifeline for those who are incarcerated, offering hope, purpose, and the opportunity for profound change.

Senghor's story shows how cultivating a love of reading can serve as a protective factor for our mental health and overall well-being. People in prison and kids who have faced abuse or neglect (sometimes both) often share a feeling that their thoughts and experiences don't matter. Research tells us that those who've been through tough times as kids may struggle with understanding and managing their emotions as adults. The effects of childhood mistreatment can lead to difficulties in thinking about and dealing with emotions.

For those in prison, who may have faced similar tough situations growing up, books become a way to connect with and make sense of their challenges. Words in these books act like witnesses to their struggles, giving them a stable reflection amid past, often unprocessed, pain. The stories within books help people in prison think compassionately about their own lives, encouraging them to understand and heal from painful experiences. In bibliotherapy, words in books become guides for a journey of personal growth—and personal growth is needed for true rehabilitation. Again, books provide a stable mirror when we are surrounded by broken glass.

TRAINING AS A BIBLIOTHERAPIST

Given the great need for empathy and connection surrounding our modern circumstances, more and more librarians, therapists, writers, and pastors (just to name a few) have been incorporating bibliotherapy into their service offerings. Unlike traditional therapeutic training that often positions the therapist as the expert, formal training in bibliotherapy diverges by emphasizing a collaborative and empowering approach, where individuals are not passive recipients but active participants in their healing journey. Some of my best bibliotherapy sessions were curated by clients themselves as they pulled from literature that elicited emotion within them and brought those excerpts and stories into session. This approach centers individuals' reading styles and preferences, centers their personhood and agency, and acknowledges the profound impact of literature in building relationships, understanding, and personal growth within the therapeutic relationship.

The International Federation of Biblio/Poetry Therapy (IFBPT) is the oldest independent credentialing organization for the profession of Biblio/Poetry Therapy and was formed in 1981. Among other training and professional community options are the International Academy for Poetry Therapy (iaPOETRY), where individuals can train as a Poetry Therapy Practitioner (PTP); the National Association for Poetry Therapy (NAPT), whose mission is to promote growth and healing through written and spoken language, symbolic expression, and story; the Therapeutic Writing Institute (TWI), which is the professional training division of the Center for Journal Therapy; and the International Expressive Arts Therapy Association (IEATA) that connects professionals from multiple fields around the concept and practice of art and expressive therapy—and these are just to name a few.

Bibliotherapists come from many different professions and walks of life. I also feel that it's important to name that anyone can incorporate bibliotherapy into their work; many of us are doing it already. In a world where we have become obsessed with credentialism and academic qualifications, we've been taught to devalue lived experience. So many brilliant minds, with so much to offer the world in terms of human potential, skill, and knowledge, are overlooked and devalued due to not being traditionally educated or trained in institutions. In writing this book, I hope to arm you with information about the field but never to discredit how much bibliotherapy has helped you or the individuals, couples, and families you serve, no matter what your education or credentials might be.

As I journey through the modality of bibliotherapy in my clinical practice, it's important to note that my own path is a testament to the accessibility of this transformative practice. Currently, I am still in the process of training to become a Certified Poetry Therapist. However, my timeline to completion remains uncertain, primarily due to the intricate interplay of systemic barriers that continue to plague credentialing programs. These hurdles are especially pronounced for individuals like me, hailing from marginalized communities with limited financial resources and support networks. The constraints of motherhood, alongside the ongoing requirements necessary to maintain my clinical licensure, further complicate this journey. It's an important reminder of the often-overlooked brilliance residing in individuals who, despite not being traditionally educated or trained within institutional systems, possess profound insights, skills, and knowledge to offer the world.

I've used this modality to help so many others, and I am still not credentialed. I want you to know this because I want you to stay encouraged and not get down on yourself by focusing too much on fancy titles and degrees. My aspiration in writing this book is to emphasize that bibliotherapy transcends conventional notions of qualification, and its impact is felt by all, irrespective of their educational background or formal credentials. You can still experience the immense power of words as witnesses, regardless of where you come from and what letters you might have after your name.

BIBLIOTHERAPEUTIC REFLECTION:

1. Reflect on the books from your childhood that left a lasting impact on your understanding of the world. How did these literary companions shape your perceptions and values?

2. Consider the significant people in your early years who introduced you to the world of literature. How did their influence contribute to your love for reading and your broader outlook on life?

3. Create a literary collage by selecting archetypes, characters, and images from the stories and fairy tales that resonated with you the most during your early years. How does the visual representation capture the essence of your inner world and the lessons learned from these tales?

PART TWO

BIBLIOTHERAPY: A DOORWAY TO INNER PEACE

CHAPTER 4

THE HOLISTIC PATH TO MENTAL WELLNESS

"I am weeping, too distraught to continue. I cannot imagine actually completing the text. Halfway through *Beloved*, Toni Morrison's meditation on the price some of us will pay to be free, I am torn asunder. Speechless, I am utterly amazed by the terrible beauty and grandeur of this tale. My tears have been shed in Auschwitz, on the Middle Passage, by rape victims, men dying in trenches, and children lit by the fires of Hiroshima. Yet in the end, the tears leave me replenished, fortified with a courage I have never known. I open the book. I can bear anything."

—MARITA GOLDEN, *The Word: Black Writers Talk About the Transformative Power of Reading and Writing*

In this chapter, we're going to explore how books can do more than just make us feel good individually; books bring people together and expand our mindsets to make us more aware of one another and more connected to each other in the social sphere. As a result of our love of literature, we gain insights into the experiences of others. Instead of thinking about wellness as something just for ourselves, we'll see how the stories we read can connect us with others and serve as windows into the world of those who have endured profound suffering. As we go through these pages, we'll discover how books have the power to build a sense of internal community and emotional wellness that comes from the awareness that we are not alone, and our experiences and inner life matter.

This chapter is all about understanding how the stories we read help shape who we are in a social sense. We'll look at how books can influence our core values and make us feel more connected to ourselves and others. To make sense of this, we'll use ideas from psychology and philosophy, like Stoicism, social cognitivism, and object relations theory. Think of it as a journey through the ways reading can make us think about ourselves and others, and how it can change the way we see well-being—as a collective rather than individual effort. We'll explore how stories, both fictional and real, have the power to transform the way we think about our mental health.

IN CONSIDERATION OF OUR SOCIAL SELVES AS READERS

I want you to think about the last book you read that made you feel seen. What was the last book you read that made you want to highlight and memorize a few lines? How about a book that opened your eyes to a different approach to a problem or a solution you hadn't considered? For me, it was *We Dare Be Brave: African American Moms and the Emotional Journey of Raising Children with Disabilities* by Salina Miller, Patricia Parker, and Charisse Montgomery.

When my son was diagnosed with autism at the height of the COVID-19 pandemic in 2020, I was overwhelmed. It wasn't because I wasn't familiar with autism. It was because I had just given birth to my daughter after the trauma of testing positive for COVID-19 in my third trimester. My husband and I temporarily moved in with his parents in South Carolina so that I could give birth with the social support of family. I can't lie, friends. I was terrified.

In March 2020, I was seven months pregnant, and my prenatal appointments were being postponed due to the panic the health care system was managing and all of the unknowns about how COVID spread at the time. I remember going to an appointment and being targeted for wearing a face mask. The supervising physician wanted to know why I was wearing a mask and if I had any symptoms. When I told her I was being safe and my toddler had a cough, she attempted to turn me away from medical care. She escorted me out of the office and asked me to leave while waving her fingers in my face and accusing me of putting everyone at risk. At this time, I was simply taking precautions. I was not COVID-positive. I was a Black mother who was pregnant while the world was navigating an unknown virus, with a—I hate to say it—white doctor screaming in my face for wearing a mask and being honest about my toddler's cough.

When I asked for documentation that she was turning me away from being seen, she paused. I very calmly (I still don't know how) and articulately (I still don't know why) told her that as a Black woman, I am very much aware of our negative outcomes with respect to maternal care. She immediately allowed me to be seen. However, I wasn't even ten minutes into my anatomy scan before she barged into the room and asked the technician if she was done. I was disgusted with the doctor's behavior and lack of empathy. With tears in my eyes, I thanked the technician for her professionalism. I looked that doctor straight in the face and told her she should be ashamed of herself for the way she treated me that day. Then I walked out of there with my head held high, knowing I did what I had to do for my baby girl's safety.

When I had my son, I was thrust into a new identity I wasn't truly prepared for. I had been grandmothered. I had never been mothered. The intensity of the parent/child bond was extremely overstimulating for me, and my son was what most nurses on the maternity floor called "colicky," a term to describe babies who cry often due to intestinal issues. I didn't know at the time that he was on the autism spectrum. So, when he was first diagnosed, I set out to find a book to mirror my experience and provide me with language and tools to navigate everything being thrown my way.

When your child is first diagnosed—and let's be honest, when you have good insurance—you are encouraged to schedule every appointment and assessment and secure every medical professional to be on your child's team: neurologist, psychologist, developmental pediatrician, speech therapist, occupational therapist, feeding therapist, nutritionist, and the list goes on and on.

Finding and reading *We Dare Be Brave* helped me navigate a sense of isolation that was pulling me under. After reading, I remember emailing Salina Miller and introducing myself and my family's story, as I was encouraged to do at the end of the book. She immediately responded, invited me to join her organization, Mother 2 Mother, and asked me what I needed and how she could support me. The authors of this book were my first Instagram live author interview. They've since become colleagues and friends. I have learned so much from these women: Black mothers on a mission to support other mothers. I would never have found community in them without picking up their book.

For parents of all children who navigate isolation and loneliness, that sense of being on your own is real. Just because people around us genuinely love us and our children doesn't mean they understand our situation or agree with our decisions. For many people, reaching out for help is very difficult. Even speaking vulnerably to a therapist can be uncomfortable, especially if you've never been supported that way before.

Incorporating a book a client loved and enjoyed into therapy helps build rapport and trust over time. Incorporating books that have impacted our clients can reveal much about how our clients show up in relationships and what they grow attached to. Literature provides a safe place to examine our values, strengths, and challenges in relationships through the lens of others. As a result, we can cope with life more gracefully and deal more creatively with what cannot be changed.

Books provide a self-paced and self-controlled way to engage in self-examination that feels less threatening than if we were to do it socially. This is important because we live our lives with our guards up to protect ourselves from the judgment of others. Sometimes, we just need to sit with ourselves and get clear about what's coming up for us without input from others.

When done in the privacy of our own spaces, reading is an insular act that grants access to our most authentic feelings. We can have a thought and understand that it is fleeting, while also holding some curiosity about what made that thought pop up for us in the first place. In my case, reading *We Dare Be Brave* provided a major mind-set shift from "What did *I do* to cause this?" to "My son is whole just the way he is because he was born this way." This was a shift from what society does to mothers—constantly judging us and nitpicking our mothering—to what mothers need to do for ourselves—honor our journeys in all their complexity and honor our children and their exact way of being in the world.

Reading provides us with a mirror to look at ourselves. Through the act of reading, we can engage with self-actualizing questions, such as: *What do I value most in the world? What am I most afraid of? Where do I find meaning, and how can I extract meaning from my life experiences?* Reading soothes our nervous system by allowing us respite from our daily realities and helping us return with more clarity, openness, and curiosity.

Have you ever read a book that immediately brought your awareness to privileges you hadn't thought of before? Maybe you read something that held up a mirror to the fact that you have a roof over your head, shoes on your feet, food on your table, a lover who is trying, or a friend who is working hard to repair the trust that's been broken. Because of generational trauma, so many of us are hardwired not to trust, or we are taught to approach life from a deficit model where we feel the need to protect ourselves from being hurt or disappointed. We cling and cleave to familiarity and would rather stay in our isolated bubble because we somehow think this will protect us.

A wise mentor once reminded me how the walls we build up to protect ourselves also keep goodness out—the goodness of being in relationship to others and developing a circle of support for ourselves, even if it's one or two loving people we can confide in. We gain self-knowledge in community with others. Learning in isolation can only take us so far. Eventually, we have to apply the knowledge that we are cultivating. The interpersonal and social rewards that a love of literature provides for us cannot be understated. We experience this in our book clubs, group chats, and social-media book communities. When we are curious about others, we are inherently self-reflective and evolving. This is good for the soul and necessary for the spirit.

EXPLORING THE INNER SYMPHONY: HOW COGNITIVISM, SOCIAL COGNITIVISM, AND STOICISM ILLUMINATE THE ROLE OF INTERNAL DIALOGUE IN SHAPING PERSPECTIVES

Stoicism, an ancient Greek philosophy, emphasizes the importance of thought awareness by encouraging us to examine our beliefs, reactions, and judgments with a critical eye. Through Stoic principles, we learn to identify irrational or harmful thoughts, paving the way for thought correction. The human mind is a maze, and thoughts enter our brains often, but that doesn't mean they are legitimate or based on truth.

The foundation of social cognitivism and Stoicism in psychology and psychiatry provides a framework for understanding human behavior and fostering mental health through literature. At the core of this framework is the ability to assess the connection of our thought life to reality. The term *thought life* refers to the continuous stream of thoughts and mental activity within an individual's mind. It encompasses the thoughts, beliefs, attitudes, and internal dialogue that shape one's perspective, influence decision-making, and contribute to emotional well-being. Cultivating a positive and mindful thought life involves being aware of and actively managing the thoughts that arise, promoting healthier mental patterns, and contributing to overall well-being. This heightened awareness facilitates a deeper understanding of our mental patterns and gives us the agency to consciously change them. An awareness of our thought life is the foundation for mental health.

Cognitivism, born out of Stoicism, underscores the significance of our thoughts, beliefs, and interpretations in shaping our psychological state. This perspective highlights the power of self-fulfilling prophecies, whereby our thoughts can influence our outcomes. We see this play out in fictional stories where self-fulfilling prophecies often manifest through a character's limiting beliefs that shape their actions and decisions. For example, is a mother who is struggling to connect to her baby a "bad mother," or is she struggling with post-partum depression? This perspective will impact the way she views her role as a mother and the support she seeks. Does a divorce mean that the years spent together in holy matrimony were not rooted in love and commitment to one another during the time things were working well? The interpretation will impact how divorced couples relate to one another and perhaps co-parent after the marriage ends. Does a friend we grow apart from over the natural course of life transitions not care for us anymore because our journeys have taken us in different directions? Our explanation will impact the way we value or devalue the time spent in that friendship. When we read, we expand our minds to consider other possibilities within our nuanced human experience, helping us make room for thought correction and self-reflection.

The evolution of psychology into social cognitivism recognizes the role of social factors, such as observation and social learning, in shaping cognition and behavior. This extension emphasizes that our direct experiences and the internalized representations of characters in literature can impact our thoughts and actions. Albert Bandura's work on vicarious learning demonstrates how we, as readers, can glean valuable insights from fictional characters, enriching our self-awareness and emotional regulation.

In practice, psychotherapy often incorporates Stoic principles and social cognitivist theories to help individuals recognize and challenge negative thought patterns. We begin to understand ourselves as part of the family of humanity. We begin to analyze the multiple roles we carry, and we get to decide what changes need to be made.

BIBLIOTHERAPY AS A PATH TO
UNDERSTANDING SOCIAL COGNITION

Reading books provides a unique avenue for self-reflection that distinguishes it from other forms of media, such as television. Reading requires an active use of our imagination. Unlike television, where visuals and sounds are provided, books demand that readers mentally construct scenes, characters, and emotions. This helps us attach emotionally to the material and allows for more profound self-reflection. We also get to control the pace of how we read and absorb information in a book. We can pause, reread, or reflect on a passage at our discretion, whereas television dictates the pace. My favorite part? Reading often stimulates our own internal dialogue. As readers, we encounter characters' thoughts and experiences in a unique way. There is no relationship in the real world where we can access someone's inner thoughts. In books, we have an opportunity to access the interiority of characters. This helps us draw meaningful parallels between a character's thoughts, feelings, and motivations and our own.

Observational learning while reading helps us gain insight into social dynamics, interpersonal relationships, and the consequences of certain behaviors. Reading allows us to identify with characters and imitate their behavior or attitudes, incorporating them into our own social repertoire. Reading fiction provides an opportunity to engage in perspective-taking by immersing ourselves in characters' experiences. We enhance our empathy and the ability to relate to diverse perspectives and social situations. We refine our schemas for understanding others.

Reading also exposes us to narratives that reflect painful social realities that may or may not impact us directly. A story's social context can influence our perception, attitude, and understanding of social phenomena in a way that feels safer than if we took those risks to connect in real life and got it wrong. Reading provides a much-needed dress rehearsal to connect to others who experience life differently than we might.

In bibliotherapy, we rely on both cognition and social cognition. Social cognition refers to the mental processes involved in how we perceive, interpret, and understand social information from our environment and use that information to interact with others effectively. It encompasses various cognitive abilities and psychological mechanisms that play a crucial role in social interactions and social behavior. Social cognition allows us to make sense of the intentions, beliefs, emotions, and behaviors of ourselves and others in social contexts.

Some key aspects of social cognition include:

- *Theory of Mind*: This refers to the ability to attribute mental states, such as beliefs, desires, intentions, and emotions, to oneself and others. It allows individuals to understand that others have thoughts and feelings that might differ from our own.

  Bibliotherapy promotes the development of theory of mind by immersing readers in the inner worlds and diverse perspectives of fictional characters. When we engage as readers with characters' thoughts, emotions, and motivations, we exercise our capacity to attribute mental states to others, fostering empathy and a deeper understanding of the complexities of human emotions and experiences. This process enhances social cognition by reinforcing the recognition that individuals, both in literature and real life, possess unique perspectives and emotions distinct from their own.

- *Emotion Recognition*: Social cognition involves the ability to accurately identify and interpret the emotions of others based on their facial expressions, body language, and vocal cues.

  Bibliotherapy enhances emotion recognition within social cognition by exposing readers to a wide range of emotional experiences through literary characters (including first-person narrators of nonfiction). When we engage with characters' emotions and their actions, we practice identifying and interpreting emotional nuances. This process strengthens our ability to recognize and empathize with others' emotions, both in fictional narratives and real-life social interactions.

- *Attribution*: People engage in attribution by assigning causes to behavior. Social cognition plays a role in how we attribute the behavior of others to internal traits (dispositional) or external circumstances (situational).

  Bibliotherapy supports the development of attribution skills within social cognition by immersing readers in complex character interactions and behaviors. As we analyze characters' actions and motivations, we practice making attributions about whether behavior arises from internal traits or external circumstances. This process fosters a deeper understanding of the complexity of human behavior and the ability to make nuanced attributions in social situations.

- *Empathy*: Empathy is the capacity to understand and share others' emotions. Social cognition helps us recognize and respond appropriately to these emotions, leading to more empathetic responses.

  Bibliotherapy is a powerful tool for enhancing empathy within social cognition by immersing readers in diverse characters' emotional experiences and perspectives. As we engage with these characters and witness their struggles and triumphs, we develop a deeper understanding of others' emotions. This process cultivates empathy, enabling readers to relate to and respond more compassionately to the emotions and experiences of real people in our lives.

- *Stereotyping and Prejudice*: Social cognition also includes how individuals categorize others into social groups and may lead to forming (and/or dismantling) stereotypes and prejudices. These cognitive processes can influence how individuals perceive and interact with people from different social groups.

Bibliotherapy is a valuable tool for addressing and mitigating stereotyping and prejudice within the realm of social cognition. By exposing readers to stories featuring diverse characters and perspectives, bibliotherapy challenges preconceived notions and encourages readers to confront and reconsider stereotypes. This process promotes a more nuanced understanding of people from different social groups, fostering empathy and dismantling prejudiced beliefs.

- *Social Decision-Making*: Social cognition plays a part in decision-making processes that involve social interactions, such as trust, cooperation, and reciprocity.

  Bibliotherapy effectively supports social decision-making within social cognition by presenting readers with scenarios and character interactions that mirror actual social dilemmas. As readers engage with these narratives, we are prompted to consider the complexities of trust, cooperation, and reciprocity in various contexts. This reflective process fosters better-informed social decision-making in readers, equipping us with insights and perspectives gained from the characters' experiences.

- *Social Influence*: Understanding the thoughts and behaviors of others through social cognition allows individuals to be influenced by others and influence others in return.

  Bibliotherapy effectively addresses social influence within social cognition by exposing readers to a wide array of character interactions and their consequences. As readers engage with these narratives, we gain insight into the ways we influence one another, positively and negatively. This enhanced understanding, empowers readers to make informed choices about the social influences in our lives, and consider the impact of our actions on others.

- *Self-Perception*: Social cognition also involves how individuals perceive themselves in relation to others, which can impact self-esteem, self-concept, and self-efficacy.

Bibliotherapy addresses self-perception within social cognition by providing readers with relatable characters and situations that prompt self-reflection. As we engage with these narratives, we often see aspects of ourselves in the characters, which can impact our self-esteem, self-concept, and self-efficacy. This process encourages a deeper exploration of one's identity and how it relates to others, fostering personal growth and self-awareness.

Social cognition is of paramount importance because it underpins our ability to navigate the web of interactions that define human existence. This complex cognitive process involves our capacity to perceive, interpret, and respond to the thoughts, feelings, intentions, and behaviors of others. Social cognition allows us to understand the perspectives of those around us and enables us to predict and influence their actions. It forms the basis for empathy, cooperation, and effective communication, all of which are vital for building and maintaining relationships, resolving conflicts, and thriving in social and professional contexts.

Social cognition is at the heart of our ability to form connections, foster collaboration, and construct the multifaceted landscape of human society. Its significance extends to virtually every aspect of our lives, influencing how we perceive ourselves and others, make decisions, and navigate the layered dynamics of our social world. Understanding social cognition also helps when picking a book that will resonate emotionally with the reader; it asks that we be culturally sensitive about what and how we read and write.

OBJECT RELATIONS AND INTERNALIZED REPRESENTATIONS

The interplay between social cognitivism, observational learning, and the enriching power of reading helps us become more aware of our thought life and, as a result, more attuned to our own mental images, which are the subjective representations we each have in our minds of experiences, relationships, and ideas. Originating from the field of psychoanalysis, object relations theory explores the complex web of our inner world and the mental representations we construct, often referred to as internal objects. These internal objects can be understood as internal images, as they are not physical entities but psychological constructs that encompass our thoughts, emotions, and perceptions of ourselves and others.

Object relations theory explores how our early experiences and relationships with primary caregivers shape these internal representations, influencing our social interactions and emotional responses. In the context of bibliotherapy, this theory invites us to examine how the characters, themes, and narratives within literature become powerful vessels for the projection and exploration of our internalized images. It can also enrich images that we never got a chance to internalize.

In her HBO special *Fighting Words,* comedian Aida Rodriguez speaks about how, through reading, she developed her concept about what a father is, what a father does, and what kind of relationship is possible between a father and a daughter. Whether you grew up with a present father or not, you soon become aware that everyone has a father, including you. So, the meaning you make out of why everyone else has a present father and you don't could be very harmful to your development. This is where core beliefs are developed, and core beliefs do not simply go away. If you were a youth who grew up without a father and perhaps developed a core belief that you are unwanted, then you will live your life believing that something is wrong with you and not the person who should be actively performing the role of father.

In her memoir *Legitimate Kid*, Rodriguez continues to express how her love of literature helped her process the traumatic events of her life: "I read one self-help book after the other. I started with *Yesterday I Cried,* followed by *Awaken the Giant Within,* and then I found another and another and kept going. Readers are leaders, Mrs. Flannagan was always in the back of my head."

When we read books, whether fiction or nonfiction, we are providing ourselves with an opportunity to develop internalized representations and working models of things we did not have growing up. We are also providing ourselves with healthier working models of things that perhaps we *did* have but that were not fully meeting our needs.

Maybe you had a parent who loved you through providing for you and doing the best they could. Perhaps that parent worked more than they were able to spend individual time with you, nurture your intelligence, and help you cultivate a sense of self-worth. This is also an opportunity for a core belief (perhaps "work is more important than other activities") to develop. But then you *read*, and you learn about the ways of the world and the inherited burdens placed upon you and your family—and you realize that your parent needing to work may not have had anything to do with you, but instead, their need to feed you and provide for you. This is an important and critical reframe that might challenge a core belief that a caregiver's absence or distance had anything to do with your worthiness.

So far, in this chapter, we have learned that reading books isn't just about enjoying stories by ourselves. It's a shared adventure that connects us with others and helps us understand ourselves and our interpersonal relationships better. These narratives are more than stories; they are compassionate companions guiding us through the complexities of life, offering profound insights into who we are and who we aspire to become.

Reflecting on my personal experience with the empowering impact of *We Dare Be Brave* while navigating the challenges of raising a child with autism, I've come to appreciate books as transformative tools that sculpt our thoughts and emotions. Drawing from psychological concepts such as Stoicism and social cognitivism, we recognize that reading isn't merely an escape; it's a therapeutic journey that shapes our cognitive landscape. Stories have the remarkable power to influence our minds, correct distorted thoughts, and heighten our emotional awareness.

In our quest for mental, spiritual, and emotional wellness, books truly become invaluable guides. They serve as mirrors, reflecting our essence and providing opportunities for gradual change. They serve as windows into the experiences of others to whom we are connected. Beyond the narrative, books offer profound lessons gleaned from characters and situations, aiding us in understanding our social relationships and self-perception. This process extends beyond the individual by fostering connections with others, expanding our perspectives, and empowering us to make informed choices.

LITERATURE AS A CATALYST FOR HEALING THROUGH MEANING-MAKING AND PERSPECTIVE EXPANSION

I am often asked, "How do therapists implement bibliotherapy into their work with clients?" The answer is simple. Bibliotherapy is implemented by recommending books, interacting with stories, and writing our own to heal. In the context of this book, healing isn't a destination proclaiming complete recovery but a continual process of integration after facing events that have fragmented our sense of self. To truly heal and restore wholeness to the self, we must process how past events impacted us. We have to make meaning out of those painful experiences. We engage in meaning-making to integrate the information we've learned about self, others, and the world into a new self-understanding and way of being in the world.

Here are some examples illustrating how reading literature helps broaden our perspective and heal from trauma while engaging in meaning-making:

Personal Reflection: After reading a novel depicting a character's journey of overcoming trauma, you might reflect on how their experiences resonate with your own. Through this introspection, you begin to make sense of your emotions and reactions, gradually integrating the insights gained from the character's story into your self-understanding. For instance, you may recognize similar patterns of coping or resilience within yourself, leading to a deeper sense of empathy and validation of your experiences.

Empathetic Understanding: As you immerse yourself in diverse narratives and perspectives through literature, you develop a broader understanding of the human experience. Reading about characters from different backgrounds and cultures allows you to empathize with their struggles and triumphs, fostering a sense of connection and shared humanity. By empathizing with fictional characters facing trauma, you cultivate empathy for yourself and others, promoting healing and compassion in your interactions with the world.

Cognitive Restructuring: Through the process of engaging with literature, you challenge and expand your existing beliefs and assumptions about trauma and resilience. As you encounter diverse narratives and alternative perspectives, you begin to reframe your understanding of trauma, moving from a sense of victimhood to one of agency and empowerment. This cognitive restructuring enables you to adopt a more adaptive way of thinking about your experiences, leading to a shift in self-perception and behavior.

Narrative Reconstruction: By reading literature that explores themes of trauma and healing, you actively participate in the construction of new narratives about your life. As you identify with characters who navigate similar challenges, you gain insights into your journey of grit and growth. Through this process of narrative reconstruction, you integrate the lessons learned from literature into your own life story, creating a narrative for yourself that reflects strength, pride in who you are, and hope.

Overall, engaging in meaning-making through literature allows you to integrate new insights and perspectives into your understanding of self, others, and the world. By actively participating in the meaning-making process, you promote healing from trauma and cultivate a deeper sense of self-awareness, empathy, and strength. For example, do I think I am fully healed from losing my grandmother at the age of fourteen? No. But I am in a state of constant recovery as I accept that healing grief is a lifelong process.

I've incorporated healing rituals that help me cope with my grief when it's activated. I tend to my emotional wounds with embodied awareness. I've read books that have helped me move through my sadness and the overwhelm of what I lost. I understand that my grandmother may not be here in the physical sense, but she is still a part of me. I derive meaning from the seeds she sowed in me that have been watered by others along my life path. I find solace in knowing that her spirit will forever watch over me, and her ancestral knowledge has become part of my way of moving through the world.

Traumatic events often leave us feeling broken, prompting the need to process their impact and derive clarity about what it all means. Healing is a practice of honoring the changes shaped by trauma, cultivating self-love, and becoming our own best friend. It's about reaching a point of self-acceptance and self-compassion where we honor our humanity and that of others. It's about being able to tolerate difficult ideas and troubling facts by consciously allowing them to be accepted without denial or repression (more on that later).

When we learn to communicate better and put our disappointments into words that enable others to see our point of view instead of internalizing pain and acting it out, that's healing. We learn to trust again and teach others how to treat us. We stop allowing the pain of past experiences to cloud the good in life and steal our joy. Books help us heal because stories offer us examples, labels, and definitions to identify and understand our emotional realities. In therapy, just as with books, we discover a space where we can be fully embraced without fear, free from the need to impress or reassure. In books, we find respite from loneliness and self-consciousness, a place where the fullness of our experiences is acknowledged.

There are three main domains where we can utilize the modality of bibliotherapy in healing therapy practice: receptive prescriptive bibliotherapy, expressive creative bibliotherapy, and symbolic ceremonial bibliotherapy. In the remaining sections, we'll cover all of these to give you an understanding of how bibliotherapy is designed to support clients' healing.

RECEPTIVE PRESCRIPTIVE BIBLIOTHERAPY

A therapist using receptive prescriptive bibliotherapy evaluates a client's present-day symptoms and recommends a book to help alleviate or reduce pain.

Receptive prescriptive bibliotherapy can either be *prescriptive* or *interactive*. When a therapist recommends a book to assist with treatment goals, this is a prescriptive action. The client can choose whether to include reflection on the text in their therapy work or simply read for personal pleasure and reflection. During interactive bibliotherapy, the client brings the selected text into the session. They may read with or apart from the therapist, using session time to reflect on the text, make meaningful connections, and deepen their understanding of their internal world. Interactive bibliotherapy involves engaging in interactive activities during a therapy session that incorporates literature as a therapeutic tool.

Here are some examples of interactive bibliotherapy in a session:

1. *Group Therapy*: The therapist may select a book or reading material that addresses specific therapeutic themes or topics. Group members can engage in guided discussions by sharing their thoughts, insights, and personal connections to the literature. This fosters open dialogue, empathy, and a sense of shared experience.

2. *Role-Playing*: The therapist and client can act out scenes or take on the roles of characters from a selected book or story. This interactive approach allows for exploring different perspectives, understanding interpersonal dynamics, and enhancing empathy and communication skills. For instance, if the book features a protagonist struggling with assertiveness, the client might role-play as the protagonist while the therapist takes on the role of a supportive friend or mentor. Through this interactive approach, the client can explore different ways of responding to challenging situations, practice assertive communication techniques, and gain insights into their behavior and emotions. Additionally, the therapist may guide clients in rewriting or reimagining the ending of a story to reflect their desired outcomes or personal growth goals. For example, if a book portrays a character overcoming adversity and finding inner strength, the therapist might encourage the client to envision themselves in a similar narrative, exploring how they can apply the character's resilience and determination to their life challenges. This exercise fosters a sense of agency and empowerment, allowing clients to reshape their narratives and cultivate hope for the future.

3. *Creative Writing*: Clients can engage in interactive writing activities inspired by literature. This can involve rewriting or expanding upon a story, writing letters to characters, or creating alternative endings. The process of writing allows for self-expression, reflection, and exploration of personal experiences. Additionally, the growing prevalence of fan-fiction websites highlights how this creative outlet can be therapeutic and foster a sense of community among writers who share similar literary interests, providing a supportive space for expression and connection. In therapy sessions, clients can participate in a creative writing activity inspired by a book they've read. For instance, if the book features a character facing a difficult decision, clients

can imagine themselves in the character's shoes and write an additional chapter exploring how they would navigate the situation. This process encourages self-reflection and allows clients to explore their values, emotions, and decision-making processes in a safe and creative way. Additionally, by sharing their writing with the therapist or fellow group members, clients can receive feedback and validation, fostering a sense of connection and community in the therapeutic space. Similarly, posting their work on fan-fiction websites provides an opportunity for clients to engage with others who share their literary interests, further enhancing their sense of belonging and support. Through creative writing, clients express themselves and find camaraderie and encouragement in their journey of self-discovery and healing.

4. *Therapeutic Games or Activities*: Therapeutic games or activities inspired by literature can be used to explore and address therapeutic goals. For example, a game may involve matching book themes with personal experiences or discussing coping strategies inspired by characters' actions. For instance, in a therapy session focused on exploring personal experiences and coping strategies, the therapist may introduce a matching game inspired by themes from a selected book. If the book revolves around themes of perseverance and overcoming obstacles, the therapist might create cards with quotes or descriptions related to these themes. The client would then match these cards with personal experiences or emotions they've encountered. As they make connections between the book's themes and their own experiences, clients have an opportunity to reflect on their strengths, challenges, and coping mechanisms. Another activity inspired by literature involves discussing coping strategies inspired by book characters' actions. For example, if the protagonist in a

book deals with adversity by practicing mindfulness or seeking support from friends, the therapist could lead a discussion on how clients can apply similar strategies to their own lives. Clients can explore the effectiveness of different coping mechanisms and brainstorm ways to incorporate them into their daily routines, which can help clients develop a personalized toolkit for managing stress and adversity.

EXPRESSIVE CREATIVE BIBLIOTHERAPY

Expressive creative bibliotherapy, which might be considered a form of interactive bibliotherapy, gives the client an opportunity to write their own story or poetry. This involves using creative and artistic activities alongside reading and writing as therapeutic tools.

Here are some examples of expressive creative bibliotherapy:

1. *Writing Prompts and Poetry*: Using writing prompts or engaging in poetry exercises can help individuals explore and express their thoughts, feelings, and experiences. In addition, creative writing can provide a cathartic expressive outlet. There are many journals and workbooks that provide readers with an opportunity to read poetry and write their own. Some of my favorites include *Healing Through Words* by Rupi Kaur and *Poetry as Spellcasting* by Tamiko Beyer, Destiny Hemphill, and Lisbeth White. *Kwame Alexander's Free Write: A Poetry Notebook* is a great option for young people.

2. *Art and Visual Expression*: Incorporating visual arts, such as drawing, painting, or collage, can complement the therapeutic process. Individuals can create artwork inspired by characters, themes, or emotions from the literature they engage with, allowing for a nonverbal expression of their inner world. This is a go-to tool for me, especially when it

comes to clients who struggle with verbal processing!

3. *Drama and Role-Playing*: Acting out scenes or engaging in role-playing activities based on characters or scenarios from books can facilitate emotional exploration and promote empathy. This approach allows individuals to step into different perspectives and gain insight into their experiences. When I worked in middle schools, I enjoyed engaging young people in creating alternative endings to stories we read in the classroom. I also loved to watch plays they would put on (shout-out to Ms. Parkins) while engaging with one another through the text.

4. *Music and Songwriting*: Integrating music and songwriting can be a powerful tool for emotional expression. Individuals can create songs inspired by book themes, characters, or personal experiences, providing an avenue for self-reflection and communication. For anyone interested in engaging young people in this intervention, I highly recommend the documentary *Stand Up & Shout: Songs from a Philly High School* from Emmy-winning filmmaker Amy Schatz.

5. *Guided Imagery*: Engaging in guided imagery exercises inspired by literature can help individuals imagine and visualize healing and transformative experiences. This technique allows them to tap into their imaginations and create mental images that promote emotional exploration and personal growth. By opening the portal of imagination, clients gain access to possibilities that would otherwise be difficult for them to consider.

6. *Journaling and Reflective Writing*: Keeping a journal to document thoughts, reflections, and insights while engaging with literature is a valuable tool for self-discovery. Writing about personal connections to the literature or reflecting on the impact of certain themes can deepen the therapeutic process.

SYMBOLIC CEREMONIAL BIBLIOTHERAPY

Symbolic ceremonial bibliotherapy involves using books or literature in a ceremonial or ritualistic manner to explore and address emotional or psychological issues. The specific rituals and practices can be tailored to individual preferences, cultural traditions, or therapeutic goals, allowing for personalized and symbolic engagement with literature. Here are a few examples:

1. *Book-Burning Ceremony*: In this symbolic ritual, individuals may choose to burn or release books that represent negative emotions, past traumas, or limiting beliefs. The act of letting go through fire symbolizes the release of emotional burdens or attachments.

2. *Book-Blessing Ritual*: This ritual involves selecting books that hold personal significance or meaning and bestowing blessings upon them. It can be done individually or as a group, where participants offer words of gratitude, intention, or affirmation for the positive impact the books have had on their lives.

3. *Reading Rituals*: A reading ritual or sacred reading group can be formed to create a safe and supportive space for individuals to explore and discuss literature that addresses personal or collective healing themes. The group may engage in specific rituals or practices, such as setting intentions before reading, sharing reflections, or incorporating meditative or contemplative practices during the reading process. One of the most profound reading rituals I've had the pleasure to participate in was organized by Indigenous Taino Cubana Juliet Diaz, who comes from a long lineage of spiritualists and brujx (a recently coined Afro-Latinx term and identity, signifying a gender-nonconforming reinterpretation of the traditional Spanish term *bruja/o*, witch or sorcerer). In response to the horrendous bombing

happening in Gaza as I write this, Juliet organized a ceremonial gathering for healers to come together. We combined literature, somatic healing, spirituality, and
inspirational messages and songs to honor our ancestors
and ask for the strength and guidance needed for the
times. I was honored to read a poem by Palestinian poet
Remi Kanazi. I could feel goosebumps as I read in community over the Zoom call. To be in the presence of so many
powerful medicine womxn reminded me of the healing
power of ritual in community.

4. *Book-Offering Ceremony*: This ceremony involves offering
   books or literary works as gifts or acts of kindness to others. The act of sharing meaningful books can symbolize
   connection, empathy, and the power of literature to inspire and uplift. Shout-out to the community book-swap
   organizers in our neighborhoods! Some of my favorites
   include The Free Black Women's Library, Norwood
   Community Library (local to the Bronx), and Blk Book
   Swap, Inc.

5. *Ritualistic Journaling with Literature*: Incorporating literature into a ritualistic journaling practice can be a form of
   symbolic ceremonial bibliotherapy. Journaling involves
   the practice of regularly writing down one's thoughts, feelings, and experiences, often as a means of self-reflection or
   documentation. Ritualistic journaling, on the other hand,
   adds a deliberate ceremonial or symbolic aspect to the process, incorporating specific rituals, prompts, or practices
   to deepen introspection and connection with oneself or
   spiritual beliefs. While traditional journaling focuses primarily on recording events and emotions, ritualistic journaling intertwines personal reflection with intentional
   acts, fostering a deeper sense of mindfulness and purpose
   in the writing process. Individuals may select passages or
   quotes from books that resonate with their personal

experiences or emotions and use them as prompts for reflection, self-exploration, or creative expression. Rituals are known to be linked to our values, making this practice a powerful means to reconnect with our sense of self and the meaningful aspects of our lives, especially during turbulent times. This structured, scheduled journaling approach enhances the therapeutic benefits and creates a space for individuals to derive comfort and meaning. This is a great way to incorporate the use of a reading journal!

CASE STUDY: PROCESSING GRIEF AND LOSS

My first time practicing bibliotherapy for personal healing was symbolic ceremonial bibliotherapy at age fourteen, when my grandmother, who raised me, passed away. This occurred at my grandmother's funeral, when I stood up and read a poem I had written for her based on her favorite Bible scripture, Psalm 23, which begins,

The Lord is my shepherd;
I shall not want.
He makes me lie down in green pastures;
he restores my soul.
He leads me beside still waters;
he leads me in paths of righteousness
for his own name's sake.

Even though I walk through the valley of the shadow of death,
I will fear no evil.
For thou art with me, O Lord;
thy rod and thy staff, they comfort me.

Through tears, deep chest breaths, and occasional sobs that I tried my darndest to hold back, I read the poem aloud as the final ritual I'd be able to perform with her physically beside me. I wanted to bless her in the words she often prayed. I wanted everyone in that room to know that while they were also grieving, my life would be fundamentally changed in a way that others would not experience. I had no home base without my grandmother. Sure, I had parents, and the family members who were under the roof of the funeral home with me, but when it all came down to the come down, my grandmother was the only person who consistently cared for me when others would not.

Not having that stable home base anymore, I did not know what would become of me or my life. The only way I could express my rage and confusion about this was in a poem I read aloud, so my pain could be witnessed by everyone in the building. After reading my poem, I folded up the verse and placed it in the palm of my grandmother's right hand before her casket was closed.

Symbolic ceremonial bibliotherapy is about meaning-making. It's about creating a ritual practice of expression we can engage in for ourselves when we are coping with major shifts along our life's journey. It wasn't until years later that I realized this was what I had done, but intuitively, some part of me understood that this symbolic act was my way of opening a window to my healing.

BIBLIOTHERAPEUTIC REFLECTION:

Let's create a simple and meaningful ritual based on what you've learned:

Self-Reflection Book Offering Ceremony

1. *Gather your books*: Begin by selecting a few books from your collection that have had a significant impact on your life emotionally, spiritually, or intellectually.
2. *Set the space*: Find a quiet and comfortable space where you can focus without distractions. Light a candle or burn some incense if you wish, creating a serene atmosphere.

3. *Reflect*: Take a few moments to reflect on the themes, messages, and experiences these books have brought into your life. Consider how they have shaped your thinking, provided comfort, or inspired you.

4. *Choose your offering*: Select one book you feel particularly connected to or that holds special significance for you. This will be the book you offer in this ceremony.

5. *Offering*: Hold the chosen book in your hands and speak aloud or silently express your gratitude for the wisdom, insights, or comfort it has provided you. Acknowledge its role in your journey and how it has enriched your life.

6. *Release*: If you feel comfortable, close your eyes and visualize releasing any negative emotions, limiting beliefs, or burdens you may be carrying. Imagine these being absorbed by the book as you offer it symbolically.

7. *Set an intention*: Set an intention for yourself moving forward. It could be a commitment to self-care, growth, or letting go of what no longer serves you.

8. *Action*: Consider taking a practical step to honor your intention. It could be journaling about your reflections, reaching out to someone, or engaging in a self-care activity.

9. *Closing*: Conclude the ritual by expressing gratitude for the opportunity to engage in this symbolic ceremony and for the wisdom gained from your books. Blow out the candle or extinguish the incense, signifying the end of the ritual.

10. *Integration*: As you go about your day, carry the intention you set with you, allowing it to guide your actions and mindset.

Remember, this ritual is about personal meaning and connection, so feel free to adapt it to suit your preferences and beliefs. The most important aspect of the ritual is to engage with sincerity and openness to the transformative power of symbolism and reflection.

CHAPTER 5

POETRY THERAPY
CAPTURING MOMENTS AND ENGAGING THE SENSES

Listen. What do you hear in your stillness? In a moment of deep feeling, what have you heard from your innermost self? Who did you turn to?

—HYEJUNG KOOK IN 'POETRY AS SPELLCASTING'
EDITED BY TAMIKO BEYER, Destiny Hemphill and Lisbeth White

We now enter the unique intervention of poetry therapy, a distinct branch of therapeutic literature. While bibliotherapy often relies on narrative structures with a clear beginning, middle, and end, poetry therapy takes a different approach. Through poetry therapy, we form deeper connections with the text and ourselves. Poetry's brevity and ambiguity invites readers to fill in the gaps with our own experiences and emotions.

As we'll explore in this chapter, poetry therapy offers a unique path to emotional catharsis and healing by capturing moments, engaging our senses, and using literary devices to reveal our inner landscapes. Unlike stories, which provide structured plots with a beginning, middle, and end, poetry allows us to sit with a moment and stay present in it. The brevity and intensity of poetry allow us to revisit and reexamine significant instances in our lives, fostering a deeper connection with ourselves and facilitating the emergence of suppressed emotions. Through the power of poetry, we can find so-lace, understanding, and healing. And the beauty of it is that two people can read the same poem and come away from it with entirely different interpretations. The heart of poetry as therapy is about what it specifically speaks to you.

Psychologist, professor, and poetry therapist Nicholas Mazza writes about the importance of asking our clients: "What does it mean for you?" Whether we are reading a poem in its entirety or simply reflecting on a stanza or choice of words, the client's interpretation of what they are reading is the most important and illuminating element in their healing practice. By inviting the client to share their personal reactions to poetry, we offer them an important element of control in the therapy room. This is a powerful tool to de-center the therapist and center the client's voice and experience (it's all about decolonizing therapy, c'mon somebody). The clinician is there to provide a sense of support and security for the client while remaining interested, first and foremost, in the client's interpretation. This approach promotes early engagement in the therapy process and fosters the client's verbalization and self-expression.

THE CASE OF ANNIE | HIP-HOP THERAPY

Hip-hop, born from the hearts and minds of some of the most marginalized communities, is an art form crafted by often unsung poets. The lyrics artists curate and the ways they perform and recite the magic of their words as testimony provide a multisensory experience that cues great opportunities for healing. I sometimes meet resistance to incorporating a poem into session, but as a bibliotherapist in the Bronx, I've never had a client say no to incorporating hip-hop lyrics that speak to them.

The impact of hip-hop lyrics as a therapeutic tool was central during my work with Annie, a fourteen-year-old youth in foster care with a history of being a flight risk. Having been shuffled between social workers, Annie harbored understandable resentment toward yet another newcomer to her life. Her journey into the foster care system commenced at the tender age of ten, marked by her parents' struggles with drug addiction and their inability to provide proper supervision.

Before Annie's case landed on my desk, she had experienced two potential adoptions that ultimately fell through, allegedly due to her perceived noncompliance with her service plan. As I embarked on getting to know Annie, her profound affinity for hip-hop was clear. She possessed an encyclopedic knowledge of Nas's lyrics from every track on the seminal album *Illmatic*. A radiant smile graced her face when she reminisced about this album's significance in connection with her father. In her cherished memories, the album served as the soundtrack to her last recollection of her father's sobriety, a time when they danced together in the living room.

Recognizing the profound emotional resonance that hip-hop held for Annie, I decided to include her passion for this art form into our therapy sessions as a poetry therapy intervention. With hopeful anticipation, I asked her to craft a haiku dedicated to her father, who was then undergoing rehabilitation. In this instance, the power of hip-hop transcended mere musical preference; it became a conduit for Annie to connect with her emotions and navigate the complexities of her past.

The prompt was: "Think about Nas's song 'It Ain't Hard to Tell' and write a haiku about what is not hard to tell for you about the truth of your life experience."

Here's what she wrote:

There's a little girl
Forced to become a woman
It ain't hard to tell

Adultification. The loss of childhood innocence. The force of life being thrust upon us, even when circumstances seem so unfair. That's what this haiku is about. I reflected to Annie that I wondered what it is like to be a young girl who feels forced into anything.

How does she manage the interruption?

How does a girl become a woman before she is ready?

How does the world treat a girl, particularly a Black girl, who navigates life with the maturity of a woman, even if it's false?

When Annie began to cry, I knew that some part of what I said, and what she wrote, was opening a gateway for her tears to flow. I sat in silence and waited until she was ready to continue our process. The silence felt like it lasted forever. In time, she began to sob, to scream, and to shout, "It's not fair!" All that was left for me to do was to hold her as she continued to release, and to let her know that I agreed.

It's not fair. No child should be forced into becoming anything or anyone. Every child deserves to go at their own pace, to be loved and provided for, to have their needs met so they can become who they are meant to be in this world. By the time our session was over, Annie had made some deep connections between being a young person in the foster care system, an African American girl in the United States raising herself, and a vulnerable youth navigating trauma.

Nas employs various metaphors in this song to emphasize his lyrical prowess and the depth of his rhymes. He compares himself to a jazz player, a wizard, and a novelist to highlight his unique talent as an emcee. In this session, Annie was able to compare herself to every other Black girl who has felt forced to reconcile the expectation of becoming a woman or being adultified long before they felt ready.

THE ESSENCE OF POETRY: CAPTURING MOMENTS

Unlike conventional books, where stories unfold over time, poetry is a snapshot of emotion, an instant frozen in words. Poetry distills complex emotions and experiences into concise verses that capture a single moment, a fleeting feeling, or a profound insight. This unique characteristic of poetry allows readers to dive deep into our emotions, revisiting and reexamining pivotal moments in our lives.

One of my favorite poems to incorporate into poetry therapy is "Diving into the Wreck" by Adrienne Rich. Rich (1929–2012) was a prominent American poet, essayist, and feminist icon whose literary contributions left an indelible mark on the landscape of twentieth-century American literature. Her style as a poet is characterized by bold and unapologetic explorations of complex themes, including gender, sexuality, politics, and identity. Rich's poetry often employs vivid and evocative language, making extensive use of metaphors and imagery to convey her ideas and emotions.

These lines always resonate with my clients, no matter what walk of life they come from:

> I came to explore the wreck.
> The words are purposes.
> The words are maps.
> I came to see the damage that was done
> and the treasures that prevail.

Doing the work of healing while self-reflecting and bringing our awareness to painful memories and experiences that have impacted us feels like exploring the wreck. This is also a great metaphor to explain why it takes time to see outcomes in psychotherapy. Where there is a wreck, there is lots of damage. There is wounding. It's best not to dig but to go slow. To sit with and observe the wreckage. To give ourselves time to process the things that will never be the same. To allow reality to settle in and grasp the helping hand that is offering some respite and assistance toward the repairs that are needed.

We cannot access words when we are in shock after a traumatic event, and we shouldn't be in a rush to. The nature of poetry therapy is to provide us with access to the moment and to the feelings that come up as a result. Then, through the poet's lens, when we are ready, willing, and able, we can begin to explore the damage at the pace that feels right for us. At this point, we can consider that even though the wreck of personal tragedy is upon us, treasure still exists in the possibility of what can be found at the site of our wounding.

ENGAGING THE SENSES:
A MULTISENSORY EXPERIENCE

Poetry transports us to the very heart of an experience. We feel the warmth of the sun on our skin, taste the salt in the sea breeze, and hear the whispers of the wind through the trees. This multisensory experience places us back in those important moments we are encouraged to recollect while reading.

Reading poetry provides a multisensory experience that has the profound capacity to connect us to our bodies and foster somatic healing. *Somatic healing* refers to a holistic approach to healing that focuses on the interconnectedness of the mind and body. It involves recognizing and addressing the physical manifestations of emotional and psychological trauma. It aims to release stored tension, promote self-awareness, and restore overall well-being. Somatic healing practices often include techniques such as body awareness, movement, breathwork, and mindfulness to facilitate the integration of emotional experiences within the body. This approach acknowledges the body's role in processing and expressing emotions, emphasizing the importance of embodied practices in the healing journey.

This concept of reading poetry as somatic healing is rooted in the idea that poetry can engage our senses in a unique way, stimulating our intellect and physical sensations. As we experience a poem, we often find ourselves conjuring images, feeling the rhythms of the verses, and even having visceral reactions to the emotions conveyed. This process deepens our connection to our physicality, grounding us in the present moment.

Somatic healing theory posits that such reconnection to our bodies is essential for improving our overall emotional and psychological well-being. When we are attuned to our bodily sensations, we become more aware of our emotions and can process them more effectively. This can lead to reduced stress and anxiety and a greater sense of inner peace, ultimately contributing to a more holistic sense of well-being. With its ability to bridge the gap between the intellectual and the sensory, reading poetry can be a potent tool for a somatic healing journey, helping us reconnect with our bodies to nurture our emotional and psychological health.

THE POWER OF LITERARY DEVICES TO TAKE US DEEPER

In poetry therapy, which encompasses the musical lyrics we take in and that transform our understanding of our lives, literary devices such as simile, metaphor, allegory, and symbolism are the therapist's tools for unlocking emotional catharsis and healing. These devices are not mere embellishments; they serve as gateways to our inner worlds.

Simile compares one thing to another, drawing parallels that invite us to see our experiences from a new perspective. For example, "My grief is like a heavy stone, sinking me into despair."

Metaphor takes this one step further, equating one thing with another to create a profound connection: "The scars of my past are a roadmap to my soul's journey."

Allegory tells stories with hidden meanings, allowing us to project our experiences onto the narrative. Allegory is a literary device employed by many writers. For example, certain stories, like C.S. Lewis's *The Chronicles of Narnia*, use biblical allegory, employing themes from the Bible to explore the battle between good and evil. For example, in Narnia, the lion Aslan is a Christ figure, sacrificing himself and then coming back to rule the kingdom. It can also mean looking at the Bible's stories in a symbolic way—which was common during the Middle Ages—rather than taking them literally. Through these hidden layers, we uncover insights about ourselves and our emotions.

Similes and metaphors allow us to bridge the gap between the familiar and the unfamiliar, enabling us to grasp and express our emotions and experiences by drawing parallels with something we already understand. With their layers of symbolism, allegories allow us to explore abstract concepts through concrete narratives, making it easier to grapple with existential questions and life's inherent challenges. In essence, these literary devices enable us to process, share, and transcend the most difficult aspects of our human existence, offering solace, insight, and the potential for healing during times of struggle.

MAKING DEEPER CONNECTIONS

In the words of author Jeanette Winterson, "Fiction and poetry are doses, medicines. What they heal is the rupture reality makes on the imagination." For some individuals, the way back to connection with imagination is easiest through a poem. Poems are usually shorter than stories yet still have such powerful stories to tell. Stories about our inner worlds and how we experience the outside world. Stories that distill the essence of our human nature into just a few lines.

Sometimes, a poem can be three lines long and pack a therapeutic punch that provides just enough enrichment to help elicit some emotion. I immediately think of Lucille Clifton's "Out of Body," where she writes: "I am saying / I am trying to say / from my mouth / but baby there is no / mouth."

As a therapist, I've witnessed the transformative power of poetry, which helps readers make meaningful connections between the symbolism in a poem and their most authentic thoughts, feelings, fears, and longings. When we can see it, hear it, taste it, touch it, and smell it, we can allow a feeling response to happen. Poetry's use of symbolism and metaphor often provides a safe opportunity for individuals to explore their inner worlds and express emotions that might be difficult to articulate otherwise. This process is especially beneficial for those from marginalized communities, who frequently don't have the luxury of time to fully engage with their emotions due to societal pressures and systemic challenges. I always tell my clients that my favorite mental health hack is carrying a book of poetry everywhere!

Poetry grants us permission to wade into our feelings but not get stuck in them. By drawing parallels between the poem's symbolism and our lives, readers can confront their emotions, fostering self-awareness, emotional release, and, ultimately, healing. Poetry therapy is a valuable tool that empowers readers to honor our own narratives and, in doing so, navigate the complex landscape of our identities and experiences.

THE FATHER OF POETRY THERAPY

During my process of writing this book, I had the honor of interviewing Nicholas Mazza. Mazza is the founding editor of the *Journal of Poetry Therapy: The Interdisciplinary Journal of Practice, Theory, Research, and Education*. In his book *Poetry Therapy: Interface of the Arts and Psychology*, Mazza writes about the theoretical foundation for the use of poetry in healing practice. Adlerian psychology encourages us to understand our clients and their inner worlds through an understanding of their social context. Gestalt therapy asks us to consider the importance of language in establishing relationships and discharging anxious, tense energy. Freudian psychology considers our unconscious and preconscious wants and needs, which a love of reading can help bring into conscious awareness.

Mazza spoke with me about the mentorship he received from Jack J. Leedy (1921–2004), a therapist and psychiatrist known as the father of poetry therapy. The director of the Poetry Therapy Center in New York City, Leedy established poetry therapy as a clinical practice in 1969 with the publication of his anthology *Poetry Therapy: The Use of Poetry in the Treatment of Emotional Disorders*.

Leedy was well-known for his saying, "Take two aspirin and one poem." That is, Leedy suggested that clients pop a couple pills and go sit and read a poem. I love that. It speaks to how painkillers can help but do not cure all the pain. Pain is expressed through intentional assertion, observation, verbalization, utterance, and explication. We express by riding the waves of emotional intensity and learning to swim rather than drown. Poems distill moments into digestible encounters that allow us to see, feel, taste, hear, and smell life again. More specifically, poetry puts us back at the scene.

Leedy wrote extensively about the *iso principle* as a key factor in choosing the right poetry to use with a client. The iso principle is a concept from music therapy that states that music (or in this case, literature) used in therapy should match the mood or "mental tempo" of the patient. Many readers instinctively use this strategy to select a new read, not finish a read (#TeamDNF), or take a break from a current one.

Leedy also encouraged his clients to write their own poetry. He stated, "Many peptic ulcers and psychosomatic ailments are poems struggling to be born." I definitely agree with this. Pain that goes unprocessed manifests in the body as physical reactions.

How many of us struggle to find a voice?

How many of us experience the voices of others as louder than our own?

Self-expression takes vulnerability and bravery, but more than anything, it takes self-possession and a desire to speak to what you feel. Once you get clear about what you have to say, you can find a way to express it. That's the power of literature to heal. The authors have already expressed what they have to say. And now, as readers, we get to take it in and digest it. If it resonates, it will teach us or remind us of something that promotes our healing. Being able to tune into our inner voice is the most important prerequisite to using it.

HIP-HOP THERAPY

The transmutative potential of poetry as a healing medium is tied to an oral storytelling tradition, where the curative properties unfold through the connection established between performers and audiences, frequently in the immersive context of large gatherings. I think about how powerful it has been in my life, for example, to see my favorite artists live in concert and the energy I carry as I leave the venue after being uplifted by the impact of their spoken words.

Few artists are as expressive and self-possessed as those in the hip-hop music genre, which we explored earlier in this chapter. One approach that draws from poetry therapy is hip-hop therapy, developed by Edgar H. Tyson (1963–2018). Hip-hop therapy is a framework focused on incorporating hip-hop lyrics and elements into mental health treatment. A creative and culturally responsive form of therapy, hip-hop therapy empowers the most historically disempowered. In the words of Shanita Hubbard, "Hip-hop was born out of a need to become a microphone for voices muted by white America."

Hip-hop therapy combines elements of hip-hop culture and music with therapeutic interventions to support healing and personal growth. It uses the power of hip-hop music, lyrics, and culture to engage individuals in self-expression, storytelling, and exploring personal narratives. Hip-hop therapy recognizes the cultural relevance and significance of hip-hop as a medium for empowerment, identity exploration, and resilience. By incorporating elements of hip-hop culture into therapy, I've been able to provide my community with a platform for personal growth, self-reflection, and social connection that resonates deeply.

Hip-hop has provided a musical form of storytelling to youth living with and navigating risk factors in the inner city for decades. Since the 1970s, hip-hop has been a way for young people to resist, revolt, express, and create amid some of the most painful life experiences and circumstances. In *A Section of My Life*, UK hip-hop artist Shocka shares his experience of being diagnosed and living with schizophrenia. He speaks to the way music and poetry have helped him cope, heal, and find community. Shocka writes: "I now know not everyone, but a majority have self-love, self-image issues and a faulty belief system. I think that was my purpose: to heal myself so I know it works, then spread the gospel to the world and teach how I did it through music and poetry."

In the same vein of self-humanizing, artist Cardi B is known for reminding fans that she'd rather not be placed on anyone's pedestal: "I'm just a regular, degular, shmegular girl from the Bronx."

The Bronx has been a significant birthplace and foundational location for hip-hop culture. Hip-hop was born in the Bronx in the 1970s to resist the city's literal burning and help poets blow off steam on the block. The saying "the Bronx is burning" is associated with the socioeconomic struggles, urban decay, and series of arsons that plagued the borough during the 1970s. High rates of poverty, unemployment, and social unrest, coupled with inadequate housing and municipal neglect, led to widespread frustration and discontent. The arson epidemic, often attributed to landlords seeking insurance payouts and residents desperate for change, further exacerbated the deteriorating conditions, highlighting the challenges the Bronx faced during this tumultuous period.

DJ Kool Herc, credited as one of the founders of hip-hop, moved to the Bronx from Jamaica in 1967, at age twelve. That summer, it was reported that 158 riots erupted across the United States due to tensions between urban communities and the police who harassed them. The power of hip-hop to raise social consciousness and support marginalized communities persists all the way into the present day in the Bronx. A number of other influential hip-hop artists have emerged from the Bronx, shaping the genre over the years:

- KRS-One—Known as The Teacha, KRS-One is a legendary rapper, producer, and one of the pioneers of hip-hop. He's been instrumental in spreading conscious and socially aware messages through his music.
- Big Punisher—A highly regarded lyricist, Big Pun is a Puerto Rican rapper who gained fame in the late 1990s. He is often celebrated for his technical skills and wordplay.
- Fat Joe—Another Puerto Rican rapper, Fat Joe is one of the most successful hip-hop artists from the Bronx. He has had numerous hit singles and has been active since the early 1990s.
- Remy Ma—An accomplished female rapper, Remy Ma has made her mark in the hip-hop industry with her strong delivery and powerful rhymes.
- Scar Lip—Sierra Lucas, better known as Scar Lip, is a Bronx rapper known for her bold style and raw delivery, showcased in tracks like "This Is New York." Her music reflects themes

of resilience and survival, resonating with audiences through her unapologetic portrayal of personal struggles.

- Slick Rick—Originally from London, Slick Rick moved to the Bronx and became a key figure in hip-hop during the 1980s. He is known for his storytelling abilities and unique flow.
- Afrika Bambaataa—Considered one of the pioneers of hip-hop, Afrika Bambaataa played a crucial role in the early development of the genre and helped spread it globally.
- Grandmaster Flash—Legendary DJ and hip-hop artist Grandmaster Flash and his group, The Furious Five, are credited with introducing innovative DJ techniques and socially conscious lyrics to the mainstream.
- Lord Finesse—An influential rapper and producer, Lord Finesse gained recognition for his smooth flow and production skills during the 1990s.
- Kool Keith—Known for his eccentric and abstract style, Kool Keith is a rapper whose impact on the hip-hop underground continues into the present day.
- Cardi B—Cardi B, born Belcalis Marlenis Almánzar, is a Grammy-winning rapper and cultural icon from the Bronx who rose to fame with her viral personality and the hit single "Bodak Yellow." Known for her outspoken nature, Cardi has become a dominant force in hip-hop with hit records like 'Invasion of Privacy' and her unfiltered authenticity.
- Ice Spice—Bronx rapper Ice Spice, born Isis Gaston, gained rapid fame in 2022 with her viral single "Munch (Feelin' U)" and is celebrated for her drill-inspired sound and catchy hooks. Her unique style and distinct curly hair have made her a standout, leading to collaborations with big names like Nicki Minaj on "Princess Diana."

Building on this legacy, JC Hall is a hip-hop therapist and school social worker in the Bronx who works at a second-chance high school where he is the hip-hop therapy studio program director. A second-chance high school typically refers to an alternative educational institution that provides opportunities for individuals who have struggled in traditional high school settings. These schools aim to offer a flexible and supportive environment, often with tailored curriculum and additional resources, to help students earn their high-school diplomas and achieve academic success despite previous challenges or setbacks.

Hall's work builds on earlier clinical examples, such as a 1997 study Tyson conducted at Miami Youth Services Center (MYSC), Inc., that sought to provide hip-hop therapy services to homeless youth navigating presenting issues of trauma, abuse, neglect, and truancy. The study results demonstrated that incorporating the clients' preferred music and own songwriting into group therapy increases overall engagement in the therapeutic process. The group could lead with their strengths and have those strengths reinforced in community.

Through hip-hop communities like those in the Bronx, people in the margins of society have a voice that lets them be heard as they simultaneously heal through artistry and building community. As a result of this musical genre, so many creatives who were previously counted out could be recognized as the poets they were and are.

SPOKEN WORD AS POETIC PERFORMANCE

Hip-hop has an illustrious history that precedes the 1970s Bronx. Poetry has always been performed in cultures across the world. The public performance of poetry—especially throughout the twentieth century among Black and Brown people in the U.S.—made it accessible and extended this expressive art into something that helped our communities transcend pain and transmute it into something that also united us around our collective joy. The history of spoken word can be traced back to ancient oral traditions, in which storytelling, poetry, and performance were integral parts of human communication. Spoken word is a vital aspect of indigenous cultures, and it continues to be an essential means of preserving and perpetuating this rich heritage, knowledge, and its many values throughout the world.

The contemporary form of spoken word as a distinct artistic expression has its roots in the African American oral tradition, particularly the Harlem Renaissance of the early twentieth century. During this time, poets such as Langston Hughes and Countee Cullen used their words to address social and racial issues, captivating audiences with their powerful delivery and poetic prowess. One of my favorite memories while conducting research for this book was reading a letter Countee Cullen wrote to Sadie P. Delaney, in which he thanked her for using his poems in her treatment of clients suffering with mental challenges. Holding that letter in my hands was a reminder of the connection and community that exists among Black creatives. It was a reminder of how we support each other when we recognize the impact of efforts to help our communities heal.

The 1960s and 1970s saw the emergence of spoken word as a political and artistic movement, with artists like The Last Poets and Gil Scott-Heron using their words to protest injustice and inspire change. Scott-Heron, a legendary poet, musician, and spoken-word artist, is known for his powerful and influential works. One of his most popular and iconic spoken-word pieces is "The Revolution Will Not Be Televised." The poem was originally released as a spoken-word track on his 1970 debut album *Small Talk at 125th and Lenox*. "The Revolution Will Not Be Televised" is a social commentary that criticizes the media, consumerism, and political apathy. The title became a rallying cry for social activism and resistance against oppressive systems. The poem's thought-provoking lyrics, along with Scott-Heron's impassioned delivery, resonated with audiences and made it a timeless anthem for the Civil Rights Movement and other social justice movements.

The piece critiques mainstream media and its inability to capture the essence of a true revolution. The lines "You will not be able to stay home, brother. You will not be able to plug in, turn on, and cop out" convey a sense of urgency, suggesting that true change requires active participation and cannot be passively consumed through television or other media. The song underscores the idea that real revolution is not a spectacle; it's a grassroots movement that happens in the streets and in the hearts and minds of people. Scott-Heron's words remind us that to be part of meaningful change, we must engage directly in the struggle for justice and not expect it to be neatly packaged and televised for our convenience.

SPOKEN WORD AS EXPRESSIVE ART AND ORAL STORYTELLING

Spoken word is an art form that grew in New York City in the 1960s as a form of poetry performed on stage. The Nuyorican Poets Café was, and still is, a site for community to gather and share poems to unite and offer strategies for community care and resistance. The Nuyorican movement was shaped by the children of Puerto Ricans who migrated to New York City in the 1940s and 1950s. This was a time of a great social justice awakening, as the island of Puerto Rico continued to be exploited by the likes of Operation Bootstrap, which provided U.S.–based companies with tax incentives to move their manufacturing businesses to the island.

In *Spoken Word: A Cultural History*, Joshua Bennett writes:

Spoken word is the Western world's oldest form of literary expression. The epic poems we are taught in school today—the Odyssey, the Iliad, and the like—were not originally conceived as written text but rather as elaborate performances, as public recitation for crowds of everyday people. Spoken word, in this sense, is where poetry as we know it begins. Oral performance precedes written mastery.

Spoken word gained further popularity in the 1980s and 1990s as a form of performance poetry, with poets like Ntozake Shange and

Amiri Baraka paving the way. Today, spoken word continues to flourish as a dynamic art form, with poets using their voices to address a wide range of social, cultural, and personal topics. It has become a platform for marginalized voices, a tool for activism, and a means of self-expression, combining the power of poetry, storytelling, and performance to captivate audiences and create meaningful connections.

Among my favorite poets is Nikki Giovanni. When I was a young girl, she represented everything I admired as she spoke her mind with little to no regard for respectability politics. *Respectability politics* refers to the belief that marginalized groups, such as Black people, can gain acceptance and equality by conforming to mainstream cultural norms and values, often at the expense of our cultural identity and heritage. Giovanni has historically argued—and she's dead right—that respectability politics is a flawed approach to achieving social progress and racial equality. She believes that embracing our cultural heritage and authenticity is essential for empowerment and creating positive change. Giovanni emphasizes the importance of self-acceptance and self-love as a means of breaking free from oppressive expectations and stereotypes.

In her poetry and writings, Giovanni highlights the strength, resilience, and beauty of Black culture and encourages us to embrace our true selves unapologetically. She's known for the way she bridges poetry and preaching with an aesthetic that appealed to the elders of our communities. Giovanni's first poetry record, the 1971 *Truth Is on Its Way*, sold more than 100,000 copies in the first six months following a free public reading she did at Canaan Baptist Church in Harlem. By blending gospel music with the secular aspect of performance poetry, Giovanni was able to use poetry therapy to unite our communities and attend to generational wounds. Placing spoken word in the center of the Black church allowed the religious and God-fearing elders of our community to respect the techniques the younger generation employed as a form of resistance, play, and self-expression.

Spoken word has always been for the people, by the people. It's a movement in which many of the most prominent figures in modern times have been BIPOC artists, including but not limited to the ranks of poets like Sonia Sanchez, J. Ivy, Nikki Giovanni, Taalam Acey, Joél Leon, Roya Marsh, and more. As a vehicle for liberatory politics, spoken word was and is about engaging everyday people in the work of healing, bonding, and creating literary art—a space to be seen and to be heard. In literature, our voices are everlasting.

NTOZAKE SHANGE TAUGHT ME

For Colored Girls Who Have Considered Suicide When the Rainbow is Enuf by Ntozake Shange is a seminal work of literature that left a permanent mark on me, but more broadly, on women of color. I was just graduating with my master of social work from Smith College in 2010 when the screen adaptation came out. I remember the wave of emotions it took me through. For the first time in a real way, I felt visible on the screen. These women were navigating depression and *talking* about it. That wasn't often the case in a world where Black women are applauded for hiding our inner struggles so well.

When the groundbreaking play that took theater and merged it with poetry, thus creating the "choreopoem," burst onto the scene in the mid-1970s, it was nothing short of revolutionary. Shange, an African American playwright and poet, fearlessly dismantled traditional theatrical structures and gave voice to the complex, often silenced experiences of Black women. *For Colored Girls* laid bare the struggles and triumphs of Black women and challenged social norms, sparking needed conversations in creative spaces about race, gender, and intersectionality. Its radical approach to storytelling reverberated through literary and theatrical spaces alike and left a major mark on Black women by reshaping the trajectory of African American literature.

Through its powerful and unapologetic verse, the book explores the myriad struggles, traumas, and resilience of Black women in

America. It speaks to the profound impact of racism and sexism and the intersectionality of these oppressions on the lives of women of color. Shange's poetic narrative provides a space for colored girls to find our voices, share our experiences, and seek healing and validation. The work's enduring legacy lies in its ability to amplify the voices of those who have been marginalized and silenced, offering solace, understanding, and a sense of community for women of color who have faced similar challenges and triumphs in their lives.

"Somebody almost walked off wid alla my stuff," from Shange's book, is a poem that resonates deeply with my clients. In this poem, Shange explores the idea of personal identity and the importance of guarding one's individuality in the face of societal pressures and expectations. She encourages Black women to be who we are and to allow the truth of our interior worlds, darkness and all, to be felt.

The metaphorical "stuff" represents a woman's self-worth, agency, and experiences, which she refuses to relinquish to others in defense of herself. Through this poem, Shange confronts the challenges that women, particularly women of color, face in a world that often seeks to diminish our worth and agency. Like so many poems that sear themselves into our memories and lead to the memorization of whole passages, it serves as a rallying cry for self-empowerment and a reminder of the importance of valuing one's identity and experiences in a society that may try to diminish us. The impact of this poem lies in its ability to resonate with Black women who have faced similar struggles, offering a sense of confirmation and strength to assert our worth and protect our "stuff" from those who would try to take it away.

BIBLIOTHERAPEUTIC REFLECTION:

1. What is it about your favorite poems, including song lyrics, that resonates deeply with you and earns them a place in your personal canon? Take a moment to reflect on the emotions they evoke, the memories they stir, and the wisdom they impart. How do these works speak to your soul

and shape your understanding of yourself and the world around you?

2. Read the following stanza from "Somebody almost walked off wid alla my stuff" by Ntozake Shange. Consider what it means to you. What emotions does this poem elicit for you about your "stuff," and what has been taken that you want to reclaim?

> /i want my own things / how I lived them/
> & give me my memories/ how I waz when I waz there/
> you cant have them or do nothing wit them/
> stealin my shit from me/ dont make it yrs/ makes it stolen/
> somebody almost run off wit alla my stuff/ & I waz standin
> there/ lookin at myself/ the whole time

3. Watch *For Colored Girls* (2010), the movie based on Ntozake Shange's play, and pay close attention to what it's like to experience the spoken word aloud. How does this activate your healing and engage your senses in a different way?

CHAPTER 6

UNLOCKING THE MIND'S REFUGE

A library is a good place to go when you feel unhappy, for there, in a book, you may find encouragement and comfort. A library is a good place to go when you feel bewildered or undecided, for there, in a book, you may have your question answered. Books are good company, in sad times and happy times, for books are people—people who have managed to stay alive by hiding between the covers of a book.

—E.B. WHITE, *Letters of Note*, 1971

In our journey toward healing and self-discovery, it's natural to seek comfort and avoid things that might hurt us. We often find peace in what is considered socially acceptable, but true growth comes when we embrace all parts of ourselves, even the ones we might think are unworthy of love.

In this chapter, we'll explore the incredible healing power of reading and the path it helps us forge toward finding inner peace—that holy grail that runs through all spiritual and personal quests. Bibliophiles know that the act of reading is tantamount to creating a safe space where judgment disappears, which helps us face our pain with gentle awareness. Together, we'll navigate through the pages of books I've used with clients to address the ways we protect ourselves—specifically, those defense mechanisms that, while trying to keep us comfortable, might have slowed our emotional growth. Through literary revelations, we can work on accepting things that are tough to face. This journey isn't just about making peace with ourselves; it's about making amends with things as they are. It's about accepting what lives outside of our control. It's about finding the strength and courage to make necessary changes where and when we can.

One of my favorite aspects of my bibliotherapy practice is using literature to support parents who don't have an opportunity for breaks from the difficult work of parenting. The reality is that our society does not support parents, especially mothers, whose labor often goes unnoticed and unappreciated. In the often-turbulent journey of raising children and balancing adult responsibilities to provide for our families, finding inner peace becomes invaluable.

E.B. White eloquently captures the essence of finding restoration through reading, portraying libraries as sanctuaries for the weary soul. As a parent who frequently visits the library for some bookish alone time, I definitely agree! For exhausted, burdened parents grappling with the absence of a true support network, literature offers more than just words on pages—it provides companionship, understanding, and the opportunity for emotional rejuvenation that can elevate our lives amid our everyday concerns.

CASE STUDY
TRUE BIZ BY SARA NOVIĆ

Suppose a client has repressed feelings of grief when struggling to accept the diagnosis of a child with a disability. Instead of recognizing and accepting these emotions within themselves, bibliotherapy provides the opportunity for them to project these feelings onto someone else (a fictional character, for example) and perceive that person as struggling to process their own grief.

I share this example with you from my bibliotherapy practice with a parent, Mia, who struggled to accept her daughter's diagnosis of hearing loss. After conducting a reading intake and assessing that bibliotherapy would be a great fit for her therapeutic goals, we read

Sara Nović's novel *True Biz* in interactive bibliotherapy sessions.

Mia self-referred to therapy. She reached out with a worried heart, grappling to understand and accept her daughter's new diagnosis. She reported symptoms indicative of depression, including a persistent feeling of sadness, disturbed sleep patterns, diminished appetite, low energy levels, and unexplained physical pain with no medical cause found by her doctor.

Mia's engagement in interactive bibliotherapy while reading *True Biz* allowed us to explore the dance of grief, projection, and eventual identification with the mother character. Here is an example of how Mia was able to access her grief through projection and, eventually, (with support from a therapist) identification with the mother of the protagonist in the story.

BIBLIOTHERAPY IN PRACTICE
USING *TRUE BIZ* BY SARA NOVIĆ

1. Have a clear outcome in mind.
   - In this case study, my goal was to help a mother access her grief and emotions regarding the recent diagnosis of her child with a disability.

2. Select a text to read for your bibliotherapy intervention.
   - You do not have to read a full text. You can choose an excerpt for a client to read and if that resonates they can choose to read the full book.
   - In order to ensure you are book matching through a trauma informed lens, you should only recommend books you have read yourself with a full understanding of your client as a reader.

3. Select a text in alignment with your client's needs, identity, and treatment goals.
   - I chose *True Biz* because it teaches so many hearing readers about the deaf community.

- The overarching message of this book is one of celebrating difference versus trying to "change" or "fix" them.
- The protagonist, Charlie, was born deaf. Instead of learning ASL, the mother pushes for a cochlear implant that doesn't work and actually puts Charlie in harm's way when it malfunctions. Charlie's dad eventually realizes their mistake as parents and signs up for ASL night classes with Charlie.
- This is a major shift in parenting from the seat of anxiety to centering connection with Charlie.

4. Ask the client what they feel.
   - After reading, ask the client if they resonate with any specific aspect (character, dialogue, setting, world view, emotion, etc.).
   - Ask the client what aspects they do not resonate with. This can also lead to further insight.

5. Integrate the information.
   - After these discussions, both you and the client can gain insight into their current emotional state.
   - Use the information to inform treatment goals and to encourage steps towards positive change.

After reading and discussing *True Biz*, Mia was able to honor grief as a natural aspect of parenting. She moved from judging grief as an inappropriate response to her child's diagnosis. She moved toward welcoming a more compassionate stance on the way every parent experiences some level of grief around who they expect their children to be versus who they are. The defense mechanism of denial often manifests in parents as they navigate the complex journey of parenthood. Fueled by the fear of being perceived as a "bad parent," caregivers may unconsciously resist acknowledging or accepting challenging aspects of their parenting experiences. The societal pressure and judgment surrounding parenting can intensify this denial, creating a protective barrier against uncomfortable truths. To maintain a positive self-image and meet societal expectations, parents may inadvertently deny or downplay difficulties, hindering their ability to seek support and address underlying issues in a healthy and constructive manner.

As a result of our work together, Mia was able to both witness and integrate her grief—a heartache she didn't realize she was carrying—into her conscious understanding of the complexity of parenting. This resulted in more peace and contentment along her emotional journey of parenting a child with hearing loss.

WHEN DEFENSE MECHANISMS
DO AND DON'T SERVE US

Defense mechanisms serve as psychological shields that we each unconsciously employ to protect ourselves from distressing or threatening thoughts, emotions, or situations. These defenses work by temporarily pushing those distressing thoughts and emotions into the recesses of our unconscious minds, providing momentary relief from immediate emotional discomfort and enabling us to navigate daily life. Additionally, they play a role in safeguarding our self-esteem and preserving our self-image; for example, to maintain a positive self-perception, we may deny aspects of ourselves that we find uncomfortable.

Let's say you have a friend who loves to snack on sweets and junk food. Even though she knows it's not the healthiest choice because she has health issues, she often tells herself, "Oh, it's just a treat once in a while—it won't hurt." She's using a defense mechanism called rationalization. It's like she's giving herself a little pep talk to justify her behavior so she doesn't have to face the fact that she might have some deeper reasons behind her eating habits, like stress or emotions she's trying to cope with.

Now, picture another friend who sometimes feels insecure about himself, especially when it comes to his abilities or how he looks compared to others. So, whenever he notices someone else's flaws or shortcomings, he quickly points them out and criticizes them. It's like he's projecting his own insecurities onto others, saying, "Hey, look at their flaws, not mine!" This way, he avoids dealing with his feelings of inadequacy and maintains an image of confidence and superiority. This defense mechanism can be seen as projection and deflection.

In both cases, these defense mechanisms are like little shields we put up to protect ourselves from facing stuff that makes us uncomfortable about ourselves. But it's important to remember that while these tricks might give us some temporary relief, they don't really help us grow or tackle the real issues at hand. So, it's all about finding a balance between being kind to ourselves and being honest about what's going on inside.

There are many other forms of defense mechanisms. Let's explore them below.

Repression: Repression helps us relegate distressing memories or emotions to the background, granting us emotional regulation and temporary respite from the intensity of life. For instance, let's say you have a family member who experienced a traumatic event in the past, such as a car accident. Whenever they think about or encounter reminders of the accident, they feel overwhelmed by fear, anxiety, and distress. It's like reliving the event all over again, and it makes it hard for them to focus on anything else or go about their daily life. To cope with these intense emotions, they unconsciously employ the defense mechanism of repression. They push the memories and associated emotions of the accident deep into their subconscious, almost like locking them away in a mental vault. By doing so, they temporarily alleviate the overwhelming feelings and regain a sense of emotional stability. With the distressing memories and emotions tucked away, they are better able to function in their daily life without constantly being haunted by the past. They might go about their routine, engage in activities they enjoy, and interact with others without the constant interference of the traumatic memories.

However, it's essential to recognize that repression provides only temporary relief. The suppressed memories and feelings are still present beneath the surface, potentially impacting their mental health in the long run. Eventually, these repressed emotions may resurface, demanding attention and resolution for them to achieve lasting healing and emotional well-being.

Humor: Humor can provide an outlet to channel our distress into more socially acceptable or constructive forms, ultimately contributing to our emotional well-being.

Imagine you know someone who recently went through a breakup. Instead of wallowing in sadness, they start making lighthearted jokes about their dating misadventures and the absurdities of relationships in general. They infuse humor into the situation as a coping mechanism to deal with their distress in a more socially acceptable way. They might crack jokes about their ex's quirky habits or poke fun at the rollercoaster of emotions that come with heartbreak. Through humor, they lighten the mood for themselves as well as those around them. This helps alleviate some of the heaviness of the breakup while allowing them to process their emotions in a healthier manner.

When we immerse ourselves in literature, we encounter characters and narratives that often reflect the complexities of human experience, including moments of hardship and adversity, through humor-infused storytelling. In fact, literature provides readers with a unique opportunity to find levity in life's challenges. For instance, witty dialogue, comical situations, and humorous characters can offer readers a refreshing perspective on their own struggles, encouraging them to approach difficulties with a sense of humor. By engaging with humorous literature, readers find temporary relief from distress and learn to navigate adversity with creativity. Whether through the absurd escapades of a comedic novel or the clever wordplay of a satirical essay, literature serves as a rich source of comedic relief, fostering emotional well-being and promoting a positive outlook on life. Here are two examples from two of my favorite texts:

1. *Their Eyes Were Watching God* by Zora Neale Hurston: "*So she offered him a seat and they made a lot of laughter out of nothing.*" While this is not at all a comedic novel, Hurston infuses her masterpiece with moments of humor and wit. Set in the early twentieth century, the novel follows the journey of Janie Crawford as she navigates love, identity, and independence in the rural South. Hurston's rich dialogue and vivid characters often bring moments of levity to the story, offering readers a glimpse into how Black communities use humor in the face of adversity. Through Janie's spirited adventures and interactions with colorful personalities, Hurston captures the joy and laughter that can coexist with life's trials and tribulations.

2. *Juliet Takes a Breath* by Gabby Rivera: "*Less than a week with the pussy lady and already you think you know everything.*" This coming-of-age novel follows Juliet Milagros Palante, a Puerto Rican lesbian from the Bronx, as she navigates her identity and relationships. Rivera infuses the narrative with humor and warmth, using Juliet's witty observations and inner monologue to lighten the heavier themes of identity, family, and self-discovery. Through Juliet's journey of self-acceptance and empowerment, Rivera celebrates the resilience and humor within Latinx communities, demonstrating how laughter can be a powerful tool for navigating life's complexities. *Juliet Takes a Breath* offers readers a refreshing and humorous exploration of intersectional identity and the search for belonging.

Sublimation: Consider a scenario where someone feels overwhelmed by anger and frustration after a disagreement with a colleague at work. Instead of lashing out or stewing in resentment, they channel that energy into a productive outlet. They decide to hit the gym with an intense workout session, pushing themselves to their physical limits. Through sublimation, they are redirecting distressing emotions into a constructive activity. As they focus on the workout, the adrenaline rush helps dissipate anger, and they emerge feeling more centered and in control. In this way, their use of sublimation helps them manage emotions effectively and contributes to their overall well-being by promoting physical health and releasing pent-up tension.

Literature also serves as a powerful medium for sublimating distressing emotions into constructive outlets. Through exploration of characters' journeys and themes of personal strength, growth, and transformation, literature inspires readers to channel their inner turmoil into creative and productive endeavors. For example, a protagonist's quest for self-discovery or their struggle to overcome obstacles can resonate deeply with readers, encouraging them to reflect on their own challenges as opportunities for growth. Readers may find clarity in writing, artistic expression, or other creative pursuits as a means of processing their emotions and finding meaning in their experiences. Through the process of sublimation, literature empowers readers to transform adversity into personal growth. This contributes to our emotional well-being in profound ways.

In bibliotherapy, the act of reading books that emotionally resonate with us plays a significant role in lowering our defenses. When we engage with literature, we are prompted to confront the truth of our feelings, even those we might usually avoid, repress, or deny. Interestingly, within the world of books, certain defense mechanisms that might prove problematic in our day-to-day lives can become invaluable tools for self-reflection and growth.

Take, for instance, the defense mechanism of projection. In literature, projection allows us to identify with fictional characters, projecting our thoughts, feelings, or motives onto them. By attributing our own undesirable qualities or impulses to these characters, we gain a safe distance from aspects of our inner lives that we find challenging or painful to acknowledge. While projection could be disastrous in real-world situations, within the context of reading, it becomes a therapeutic mechanism for exploring and understanding our psyche.

However, it's important to note that defense mechanisms can become problematic when *not* acknowledged. This is where bibliotherapy with a trained mental health professional can be supportive to a reader's healing process. Overreliance on defenses may impede personal growth and hinder emotional authenticity. The goal of bibliotherapy mirrors that of psychotherapy: to allow our most authentic selves to emerge by becoming aware of and addressing our defenses. By engaging in adaptive coping strategies like reading and expressive writing, we can strike a balance between using defense mechanisms and exploring healthier ways of coping with distress.

THE SHADOW SELF

In addition to exploring defense mechanisms, another important aspect of understanding our inner life includes understanding the concept of the shadow self. A term coined by Carl Jung, the shadow self encompasses hidden aspects of our personality that we often suppress or deny. These hidden facets, including our insecurities, repressed emotions, and unresolved traumas, lurk in the shadows of our unconscious, exerting a subtle yet profound influence on our thoughts and actions.

The shadow self is the part of ourselves that we ignore. The part of us that contains the feelings we feel yucky about having in the first place. The part of us that can be judgmental, dismissive, envious, and even hateful. The part of us that also has something important worth expressing that we might be afraid to tune into for fear of what it all means. But feelings don't make any definite conclusion true. Feelings are simply information; by acknowledging all of them, we can engage with life's ailments with greater clarity and self-compassion.

As we navigate the landscape of our psyche through the lens of bibliotherapy and self-reflection, we inevitably encounter the shadow self. Just as literature serves as a mirror reflecting our defenses and coping mechanisms, it also illuminates the shadowy recesses of our inner world, inviting us to confront and integrate these disowned aspects of ourselves.

One important way literature helps us heal is by introducing us to the shadow self in greater depth. A love of reading supports us in acknowledging and embracing these hidden dimensions. Reading and expressive writing offer us a transformative portal to confront and embrace our shadow self. Through this process, we begin to recognize our defense mechanisms. In doing so, we gain tools and insights to explore healthier ways of coping with distress. Through this process, we honor that our shadow self exists for a reason, was born out of conflict, and has helped us survive thus far on our life's journey. By paying more attention to this part of ourselves, we come to heal and integrate all of who we are into our way of being in the world, without shame or self-judgment.

SHADOW LESSONS FROM TWO POPULAR PROTAGONISTS AT LITERAPY NYC

Edie, the self-destructive character from Raven Leilani's *Luster*, emerges as a striking embodiment of the shadow self. Edie is a young woman stumbling through her twenties in Bushwick—navigating an unsatisfying job, inappropriate sexual choices, and a simmering artistic talent. Her encounter with Eric, a man in an open marriage, catapults her into a journey of self-discovery amid contemporary respectability and racial politics. As readers are taken on Edie's tumultuous journey, we are compelled to confront our own shadow selves. Edie's reckless self-abandonment, her penchant for seeking comfort in the arms of those who may inflict harm, and her relentless self-sabotage all serve as a mirror through which readers are forced to gaze at their own vulnerabilities and inner demons. Through Edie, we are challenged to explore the facets of our psyche that may shy away from the harsh light of introspection, pushing us to question the boundaries of our own self-destructive tendencies.

Similarly, in Candice Carty-Williams' *Queenie*, the eponymous protagonist, Queenie, takes center stage as she navigates a tumultuous journey through self-abandonment and turbulent relationships. Queenie Jenkins is a twenty-five-year-old Jamaican British woman living in London, navigating the complexities of straddling two cultures and feeling out of place in both. Working at a national newspaper, she grapples with comparisons to her white middle-class peers and seeks validation in unhealthy relationships after a messy breakup, prompting her to question her identity and desires in a world that constantly imposes its expectations on her. Queenie's impulsive decisions, her yearning for affection in all the wrong places, and her constant dismissal of self-worth resonate deeply with readers. Just as Edie does, Queenie forces us to examine the ways we may neglect our well-being and indiscriminately chase fleeting connections in our search for acceptance and love. Through her experiences, we are invited to scrutinize our own tendencies, which may include self-neglect and the erosion of our intuition.

From a therapist's perspective, both stories are powerful tools for supporting self-understanding, enhancing reality orientation, and increasing awareness of interpersonal relationships. By engaging with their stories, clients can uncover parallels in their lives, providing opportunities for meaningful exploration and growth. These characters serve as catalysts for therapeutic discussions, encouraging clients to enrich their internal images and develop healthier coping mechanisms.

I had one client exclaim during a session, "Edie really needed some homegirls to tell her she was trippin'!" And she was right! Through the therapeutic lens of literature, clients can readily identify growth areas, ultimately finding the strength to confront their shadow selves, needs that have gone unmet, and authentic feelings that arise. Then, they can chart a path toward healing and self-fulfillment.

There is no place I have found more amenable to meeting my shadow self than within the pages of a great book. While reading, I can judge without being judged. I've learned quite a lot about myself while engaging in literary escapism. In reading to mentally escape from the realities of everyday life, I've been pleasantly surprised to find the most authentic version of myself looking back at me. Books are a place where the less desirable thoughts and feelings I've had have been able to engage in dialogue with me, reflecting back hard truths that have been difficult to accept in my daily life.

BIBLIOTHERAPEUTIC REFLECTION:

1. Think of a fictional character that activated your frustration or disappointment. What was it about them that activated you?
2. Are any of the qualities you despised in them qualities you can identify in your shadow self?
3. How can embracing the parts of yourself that you are ashamed of lead to healthier coping skills that actually soothe you and reduce self-judgment?

PART THREE

BIBLIOTHERAPY AS A PATH TO COLLECTIVE WELL-BEING

CHAPTER 7

EMBRACING STORIES OF TRAUMA AND HEALING

READING AS EMPATHY AND CONNECTION

A great deal of psychology focuses on the individual, but for emotions this is not ideal. Although we experience emotions personally, most of them are interpersonal.

—KEITH OATLEY, *Our Minds, Our Selves: A Brief History of Psychology*

In the final part of this book, we will discuss the intergenerational power of reading as a tool for healing, allowing us to connect with the struggles and triumphs of those who came before us. By embracing these narratives, we pave the way for a more empathetic and inclusive society, fostering healing on individual and societal levels alike. Literature has long been used as a healing balm to soothe our pain and validate difficult aspects of the human experience that apply to us all. Literature reminds us that, as different as we may be, the human experience makes us more alike than different.

However, one factor that makes a shared understanding of our human condition difficult is the impact of book banning on our emotional and collective landscapes. While exploring the profound impact of literature on mental health, it becomes evident that the banning of books transcends mere censorship—it is a serious community mental health issue. Literature serves as a potent tool for healing, acting as a bridge between individuals by offering validation and expanding our awareness of the human experience. When marginalized voices are silenced through book bans, we perpetuate a collective shadow that seeks to suppress the experiences of the most vulnerable among us.

In the 2022–23 school year, it was deeply troubling to note that PEN America recorded a significant 3,362 instances of book bans. These bans encompassed a wide array of works, from those tackling issues of racial inequality and LGBTQ+ themes to timeless classics like *The Great Gatsby* and *Moby Dick*. As a therapist, I see these book bans as not just acts of censorship but barriers to mental health and healing. Books play a crucial role in providing individuals with avenues for understanding, empathy, and connection. When certain perspectives are silenced, readers are deprived of the opportunity to explore diverse experiences and engage in meaningful self-reflection. It is my belief that everyone, especially students, should have access to literature that reflects the richness and complexity of the human experience. As therapists, we stand in solidarity with educators, librarians, and readers alike, advocating for the preservation of diverse voices and perspectives in literature. By fostering a culture of inclusivity and openness, we create spaces of solace, validation, and growth through the power of storytelling.

FROM CELL TO CATALYST: SENGHOR'S JOURNEY OF REDEMPTION THROUGH LITERATURE AND READING

The redemption narrative is one of the most important methods of catalyzing the kind of empathy and understanding that could effect widespread social change, given its capacity to change hearts and minds. Everyone loves a good redemption story, perhaps because it helps us uncover one of the deepest desires we have: true belonging.

One of my favorite authors, mentioned earlier in this book, is Shaka Senghor, a dynamic leader whose journey embodies resilience, redemption, and social impact. Formerly incarcerated, Senghor's transformation is a testament to the power of second chances.

As a former MIT Media Lab Director's Fellow and recipient of prestigious awards like the Black Male Engagement (BMe) Leadership Award, he is a recognized thought leader. In his work, he shares his journey of redemption and transformation with global audiences, teaching at institutions like the University of Michigan. Senghor's focus now lies in creating impactful content that combines social significance with entertainment value, aiming to shift societal narratives. Through his work, Senghor inspires us to believe in the power of resilience, redemption, and meaningful change.

In *Letters to the Sons of Society: A Father's Invitation to Love, Honesty, and Freedom*, Senghor writes a letter to his son, Sekou. He recalls the trauma of spending so many years of his prison sentence in solitary confinement. He writes that for five days a week, spanning several years, he was only allowed to leave his cell for one hour a day. It was reading that kept him grounded when he felt he was going insane from the solitude and isolation. In an Instagram post published October 6, 2023, Senghor writes: "Here is why they are banning my book 'Writing My Wrongs' in prisons. They claim the content can be used to facilitate criminal activity, including descriptions of how prisoner groups are organized and motivated to use violence and intimidation to control prisoners, financial and other unapproved activities within the prison."

Those who claim that Senghor's book should be banned in prisons because it might facilitate criminal activity are missing the point— whether willfully or unintentionally. Senghor's memoir primarily focuses on his personal journey of redemption and transformation, detailing his experiences with incarceration and the process of self-discovery. While the book touches on the realities of prison life, including the challenges and dangers inmates face, it does not provide detailed instructions or encouragement of criminal behavior. Instead, it offers insight into the human condition and the possibilities that exist for personal growth despite one's past, making it a valuable resource for rehabilitation and introspection within correctional facilities.

Senghor, now a free man, uses his platform to share his testimony of life after prison and speaks openly about how cultivating a love of reading helped him heal and stay grounded, even when his reality was too painful to bear. He quotes an excerpt from Anne Frank's *The Diary of a Young Girl* that supported him to make it through his despair. Reading Anne Frank reminded him that others have had to navigate similar dark paths. Therefore, so could he.

In *Letters to the Sons of Society*, he writes: "Reading Anne Frank, it's amazing to think that though our outward experiences were so different and took place at such different times in history, our shared sense of despair makes us siblings in pain. This is what isolation does: it creates a family." I would add that this is what bibliotherapy does: It creates connection where before there was only the sting of loneliness, providing us with validation, an expanded perspective, and new understanding. This can be particularly supportive for those grappling with depression and suicidal ideation, struggles that are often shrouded in secrecy due to shame. Validation through the recognition of shared experiences can serve as a powerful reminder of the universality of human experience and the possibility of recovery and healing—just like it did for my client Sarah.

CASE STUDY | THE CASE OF SARAH

When I first met Sarah, a seventeen-year-old high school student, she came to therapy in a state of despair. She was grappling with thoughts of suicide and a profound sense of isolation. She had faced significant trauma and adversity in her young life, leaving her feeling overwhelmed and hopeless. Sarah's journey toward healing took a remarkable turn when she read the banned book *The Perks of Being a Wallflower* by Stephen Chbosky. At the recommendation of a supportive teacher, Sarah embarked on a journey with this novel that would ultimately save her life.

I asked her to pull some quotes from the book for me so that I could better understand how this story supported her not to unalive herself. Among her favorite quotes was this one: "This moment will just be another story someday." She spoke with me about how this quote reminded her that nothing in life is permanent, not even hopelessness.

Sarah's therapy incorporated a trauma-informed approach, recognizing the depth of her emotional pain and the need for a safe and empathetic space to explore her feelings. The therapeutic process focused on resilience-building and fostering hope through literature. Sarah's experience with *The Perks of Being a Wallflower* was nothing short of transformative in the way it motivated her to stay alive and imagine a brighter future for herself.

The novel's protagonist, Charlie, grapples with trauma, depression, and alienation—themes that closely mirrored Sarah's struggles. Sarah identified with the character's emotions and the challenges he faces. She found inner peace in the realization that she was not alone in her pain. The book's narrative of healing, growth, and the power of friendship provided a lifeline for Sarah. Through Charlie's journey, she began to envision the possibility of her own recovery and renewal. Within the pages of this banned book, Sarah found a source of hope that had eluded her for so long.

Chbosky's book has faced challenges and bans in some school districts due to its explicit content, including references to drugs, alcohol, and sexual themes, which some educators and parents find inappropriate for young readers. The novel addresses issues of mental health, abuse, and homosexuality, making it a target for censorship in certain conservative communities.

Nevertheless, Sarah's experience with *The Perks of Being a Wallflower* marked a turning point in her life. The novel helped her recognize that her trauma did not have to define her and that there existed a path to healing and recovery. Over time, Sarah's therapy incorporated discussions about the book, allowing her to process her emotions and draw parallels between her own journey and Charlie's.

She started to open up to new friendships and developed healthy coping skills to manage her anxiety and depression when they arose.

Sarah's story exemplifies the life-changing power of literature, especially trauma-informed fiction. Banned books like *The Perks of Being a Wallflower* provide a platform for readers to explore their pain and discover a renewed sense of hope. Through the therapeutic integration of literature addressing painful themes, individuals like Sarah can heal, cultivate resourcefulness, and move forward with optimism.

Books that are frequently banned tend to be those that bravely confront the lasting impacts of trauma on individuals and society, offering profound insights into the human condition. By addressing themes of abuse, discrimination, mental health challenges, and other painful experiences, these books serve as vital resources for readers seeking understanding and validation of their struggles. Banning such literature stifles meaningful conversations about trauma and denies readers the opportunity for healing and empowerment through shared narratives of resilience and survival. Trauma-informed literature helps readers understand that, while painful events change us, we can transcend pain and evolve into the best versions of ourselves based on the lessons life has taught us.

TRAUMA-INFORMED LITERATURE

Trauma-informed literature provides a special kind of storytelling that focuses on showing how difficult experiences affect people's lives. It goes beyond simply talking about the bad things that happened and explores how these experiences can have a lasting impact on a person's thoughts and ways of navigating the world.

Authors who write through a trauma-informed lens spend time researching and talking to people who have gone through similar experiences to make sure they tell the story accurately and respectfully. The main goals of trauma-informed stories are not only to entertain but to help readers understand the nature of trauma healing and the way these painful experiences leave us forever changed. These narratives provide imperfect but hopeful, honest endings. They make no promises that everything will be all right, but they remind us that events that harm us are survivable, for the most part, with the right kinds of support.

It is a labor of love to write down a trauma-informed story, no matter the genre. Nonfiction, fictionalized true stories—all stories can be written in a way that leaves the reader with hopeful possibilities. This is crucial when choosing literature for bibliotherapy with a client. Trauma-informed storytelling aims to depict traumatic experiences with compassion and seeks to reflect the psychological and emotional aftereffects trauma can have on survivors, families, and communities at large. Trauma-sensitive authors typically engage with the communities they are writing about and hire beta readers and sensitivity readers to obtain feedback. Despite potentially triggering themes, a careful and sensitive approach to storytelling renders trauma-informed literature responsive to the reader's needs.

Memoirs, which are especially common in trauma-informed literature, serve as powerful tools for readers seeking healing and the opportunity to rewrite their narratives. Sometimes, we just need to see that we aren't the only ones who have gone through specific challenges. Discovering our experiences mirrored in other people's accounts fosters a sense of connection and understanding. We stop judging ourselves, and we honor the messiness of life and being human. Even the most challenging stories can be life-changing for the better. Through someone else's journey, readers may find clarity, resonance, and the inspiration to navigate their hardships with renewed hope.

THE UPCYCLED SELF

The memoir *The Upcycled Self* by Tariq Trotter (widely known as the hip-hop artist Black Thought) introduces the concept of the upcycle—a profound philosophy of constant reinvention in the face of life's adversities. The memoir serves as a testament to life after death, suggesting that even in the aftermath of personal devastation, individuals can rebuild and create something entirely new. As Trotter shares his journey, readers are invited to consider our own stories through the lens of possibility, encouraging us to view our traumas not as fixed wounds but as opportunities for growth and reconstruction. Especially for his loyal fans, Trotter's memoir becomes a guide for readers seeking healing and a blueprint for crafting new narratives from the broken pieces of their lives.

The trauma-healing journey portrayed in *The Upcycled Self* illustrates how we can gather the broken pieces of our hearts to create something meaningful. Trotter shares the intimate details of his life, recounting a pivotal moment as a young boy in Philadelphia when he mistakenly burned down his family home at the tender age of six. However, rather than dwelling on the devastation, Trotter introduces the concept of the upcycle—a way of life that embraces constant evolution through inevitable challenges.

His words echo with a profound message: "Things might be lost forever, but even when our souls are broken, burned, or misplaced, they can be rebuilt, pieced back together, quilted into something new, maybe something beautiful." Trotter's memoir is not just a recounting of personal struggles; it is a testament to perseverance, encouraging readers to view their traumas as opportunities for growth and evolution.

Trotter's impactful storytelling transcends the boundaries of hip-hop, resonating deeply with fans who admire his musical prowess as well as the vulnerability and strength woven into his life narrative. Given his deeply private nature, his decision to share his story holds even greater significance for his fans.

Reading about his mother's compassionate and loving response when he accidentally burned down the house as a child evokes powerful emotions in clients. As they reflect on this example of maternal warmth and support, clients contrast it with their own experiences, particularly if they didn't receive the nurturing they needed from their mothers. This exploration can lead to deeper insights into their emotional needs and the impact of early relationships on their sense of security and self-worth. Through *The Upcycled Self*, Trotter becomes more than a hip-hop legend—he becomes a literary guide.

TRAUMA-INFORMED ROMANCE

Our early attachment experiences with caregivers deeply shape the way we engage in romantic relationships, often leading to the reenactment of unresolved traumas. My client Ciara grew up in a household where her parents were emotionally distant and inconsistent in their responses to her needs. As a result, she developed an anxious attachment style, constantly seeking reassurance and validation from her romantic partners. Despite their best efforts, Ciara's partners often feel overwhelmed by her neediness, leading to conflict and distance in the relationship. Through therapy, she has learned to recognize the connection between her childhood experiences and her relationship patterns, allowing her to work through her attachment issues and cultivate healthier, more fulfilling connections in her adult life.

My client Alex's parents divorced when he was young, and he was mostly raised by his mother, who grappled with depression and alcoholism. Growing up, Alex felt neglected and emotionally abandoned, leading him to develop an avoidant attachment style. In his romantic relationships, Alex finds it challenging to trust and open up to others, fearing vulnerability and intimacy. Despite genuinely caring for his partners, Alex often withdraws emotionally, unable to fully commit or express his feelings. Through therapy, Alex explores the connection between his early experiences of loss and neglect and his avoidant relationship patterns, working toward healing his attachment wounds and building healthier connections based on trust and intimacy.

Romance books written from a trauma-informed lens authentically portray the complexities of trauma healing within interpersonal relationships and provide possibilities for genuine healing. We get to experience the story while observing the inner lives of characters, their relational choices, and the consequences of their behaviors and actions on others. Relationships are hard work and require us to be authentic, vulnerable, and open to growth. Trauma-informed romance stories offer hope through plots that reflect the struggle, beauty, and grace inherent in the process of loving and being loved by someone. While these books may not provide easy answers about relational repair, they validate the challenges of navigating intimacy in the aftermath of trauma, emphasizing the resilience and growth that can emerge from facing adversity together.

Before I Let Go by Kennedy Ryan is an important story in the romance genre. Ryan is acclaimed for her adept portrayal of emotionally charged narratives and her exploration of complex social issues within the genre. Unlike conventional romance narratives that may overlook or glamorize unhealthy dynamics, Ryan's approach honestly explores trauma and its impact on relationships. By prioritizing empathy and understanding, her narratives provide readers with a nuanced perspective on love, resilience, and healing. For individuals seeking a more insightful and compassionate portrayal of relationships, *Before I Let Go* offers a compelling exploration of these themes within a fictional but highly realistic context.

The novel's protagonists, Yasmen and Josiah, work toward relational repair after the loss of their infant child. The couple has two older children and run a popular restaurant together. Their lives are intimately connected through parenthood, grief, and running a business. There is nowhere to hide for these two, and although they are divorced, they must reckon with the unaddressed pain they are holding while co-parenting and living life.

This is a great book to help clients experience emotional catharsis because it shows how the trauma of loss impacts us on an often-unconscious level. Just because we do not speak about our pain or share that we are in pain doesn't make the pain go away—and that pain continues to influence our behavior. Ryan shows us how this pain impacts each member of the family and is honest about what true relational repair will require.

The ending is realistic and hopeful, and Ryan still manages to make it romantic for her readers. Couples go through hardships every day, and part of an emotionally honest love story is accepting the truth that we cannot save our partners from taking the hits that life will inevitably deal them. Likewise, we cannot control what life will bring our way when we are navigating being in a couple. The romance in this story is the glue that holds together two people who fundamentally love each other. Even when life events tear them apart, the two of them are able to find their way back to one another through healing and acknowledging their individual and collective wounds.

Ryan is beloved in the book community as an author who focuses on building real relationships with her readers. She brings that same level of attunement to her craft as a storyteller. She often speaks about her process of writing *Before I Let Go*, which centers Black love. Before writing it, she spoke with caregivers who had experienced child loss and therapists who work with grieving caregivers. Ryan conceived of Yasmen and Josiah as two complex characters who are not saved from their pain in the end, but accept their loss and move toward the possibility of a new kind of life and a new kind of love that includes their lived experience of loss. Trauma-informed stories do not promise that all will end well. They are honest about the role we must play in our own healing. Sometimes, the best endings are new beginnings.

Before I Let Go also offers readers an opportunity to understand how unhealed emotional wounds get passed down generationally in family systems, which can impact families and communities. Ryan's portrayal of the effects of traumatic child loss on the family system is meticulous, revealing its impact on all relationships. The story explores the repercussions on Yasmen and Josiah's connections with their children, friends, and therapists, offering a powerful reflection of how unhealed wounds can perpetuate the cycle of trauma. By bringing these effects to light, the author emphasizes that unacknowledged pain does not vanish and can have far-reaching consequences, echoing throughout generations. I also love that this narrative celebrates Josiah's transformative healing journey as a Black man seeking mental health support. His decision to finally attend therapy, despite avoiding it after the loss of their baby, demonstrates the direct positive impact therapy has on his ability to eventually articulate his emotions and unmet needs.

TRAUMA-INFORMED INSIGHTS:
UNVEILING THE CRAFT THROUGH *BEFORE I LET GO*

Through carefully selected quotes from the book, I aim to show you essential elements that contribute to the genre's sensitivity and empathy. *Before I Let Go* captures the essence of compelling storytelling and also addresses crucial therapeutic goals. Each quote serves as a narrative tool, guiding readers through the complexities of mental health, decision-making, relationships, and societal pressures.

Together, we'll examine how these excerpts align with trauma-informed principles, offering insights into the delicate craft of creating fiction that fosters emotional exploration and healing.

1. Goal: Increase the client's self-understanding.

This happens, Yasmen. Depression is an altered state of mind. Not just feeling sad, but the chemistry of your brain, your hormones. Your body is a participant, held hostage to depression just as much as your mind.

The quote addresses the goal of increasing self-understanding by specifically explaining the nature of depression. It serves as a therapeutic tool to educate individuals about the biological aspects of mental health, helping them comprehend the connection between their emotional states and physiological responses.

2. Goal: Improve the client's reality orientation.

> *"They talked to a survivor and you know what he said?" She pauses, waiting for me to shake my head, breath bated. "As soon as he jumped, he changed his mind."*

This quote contributes to the goal of improving reality orientation by presenting a poignant scenario that challenges perceptions. By presenting a scenario where a survivor expresses regret immediately after taking irreversible action, the quote challenges perceptions and prompts readers to confront the complexity of human decision-making in difficult circumstances. It underscores the finality of such actions, driving home the sobering reality of their irreversible consequences.

3. Goal: Improve the capacity to respond by enriching internal images and allowing emotions about those images to surface.

> *"If this is something you want," Dr. Musa says, "and you obviously have very strong feelings for her, lay some ground rules. Agree on your expectations. Articulate what you think this relationship will give you both, what you want from it, what's acceptable, the grounds for ending it. All of it. Be up front and protect both of you in the long run. If you want it as badly as you seem to . . ."*

The quote underscores the importance of clear communication and setting boundaries in relationships, a task that can be particularly challenging for men due to social norms and expectations surrounding masculinity. Men are often socialized to suppress emotions and prioritize stoicism, making it difficult to navigate and express their feelings effectively. However, by encouraging open dialogue and the articulation of expectations, desires, and limits, the quoted dialogue provides a framework for men to overcome these barriers and engage in healthy communication within their relationships. It acknowledges the unique challenges men may face in expressing emotions and offers guidance on how to navigate these complexities while fostering emotional growth and connection.

4. Goal: Increase awareness of interpersonal relationships.

"Women of color are regularly praised for our resilience, but what's too often overlooked is that our resilience is a response to so many forms of violence. For us, resilience is more than a noble trait; it's a lifestyle that oppression has demanded of us. Either we adapt or we die."

This quote addresses the goal of increasing awareness of interpersonal relationships by shedding light on the unique challenges faced by women of color. It serves to help readers explore the social dynamics influencing their lives, promoting a deeper understanding of resilience as both a strength and a response to systemic adversities.

In crafting trauma-informed fiction, authors navigate delicate themes with empathy and sensitivity, recognizing the potential impact on readers' emotional well-being. The quotes from *Before I Let Go* exemplify aspects of trauma-informed writing by providing nuanced perspectives on mental health, decision-making, relationships, and societal expectations. The narrative doesn't merely depict trauma but aims to guide readers through self-reflection and understanding. Trauma-informed fiction prioritizes authenticity, ensuring characters and their experiences resonate with readers while fostering an environment for emotional exploration and healing. It emphasizes the importance of portraying growth in relationships through forgiveness and repair, acknowledging the lived experiences of others, and creating narratives that encourage empathy and awareness.

BOOKISH JOY AS A COPING SKILL

The remedy that reading provides lies in not letting pain define our entire identity. The remedy resides in discovering how to navigate the spectrum of our emotions, including prioritizing and centering joy, peace, and presence. We must recognize our inherent right to respond to life's impact on us—period. We are all travelers on this human journey. My experience as a bibliotherapist in the Bronx has reinforced the notion that joy is not confined to specific circumstances; it can be found anywhere if we actively seek it. Our community has always understood joy as more than a fleeting state of being. Joy is a profound *understanding*—an acknowledgment that life can shift unexpectedly, whether through loss, illness, upheaval, or even minor inconveniences. Therefore, I diligently cultivate my capacity to embody joy, knowing that she resides within me, waiting to be found every time and at any time. When I write my own poetry, I like to remind myself of the importance of holding joy close to me:

> *Joy allows me to be my most authentic self in every present*
> *   moment.*
> *She allows me to close my eyes. Rest for the weary.*
> *She reminds me to savor a breath of fresh air as I open a window.*
> *She reminds me.*
> *Let me grant myself the space to feel vulnerable, whether in body*
> *   or in mind.*
> *I am human, entitled to my emotions, and still, I breathe.*
> *Joy won't allow me to abandon my breath.*

Holding tight to joy is about extending the same kindness to ourselves that we readily offer to others. It's about embracing our vulnerabilities and recognizing that there are diverse ways to engage with life's challenges, beyond constant battle. There is strength in my silence. There is strength in my stillness. There is strength in my softness. In every intentional way I choose to move forward, there is strength in my choice.

NARRATIVE THERAPY

Narrative therapy, in particular, is an approach that empowers clients to recognize their agency as the protagonist of their own life stories, affirming that strength resides in our intentional choices. At its core, narrative therapy recognizes that our experiences are woven together by the narratives we construct, both individually and collectively. Just as in the therapeutic process, where clients are encouraged to explore alternative narratives to reframe their challenges and experiences, literature provides a similar avenue for readers to navigate human emotions and conflicts. This newfound self-awareness often leads to the resolution of internal and external conflicts, because literature serves as a mirror reflecting the many dimensions of the human condition and the myriad ways in which individuals navigate our own narratives. In essence, narrative therapy and bibliotherapy converge in their capacity to empower individuals to rewrite our stories and access personal growth, inner-standing, and conflict resolution.

Narrative therapy, pioneered by David Epston and Michael White in the 1980s, offers a storytelling approach to working with clients and helping them resolve inner conflict. Narrative therapy asks us to consider the stories we tell ourselves about ourselves and determine if those stories were inherited. While narrative therapy is a distinct modality from bibliotherapy, I enjoy merging the two in my work with clients. Narrative therapy helps clients look at the multiple storylines intersecting in our lives so we can make meaning out of those experiences. A core principle of this approach is that "the problem is the problem, and the person is not the problem." In narrative therapy, the problem the client is struggling with is viewed as separate from the person's identity. For example, viewing your depression as separate from your overall identity allows you to rethink its impact on your life.

In this approach, we honor that our realities are socially constructed through our interactions with others, the way we experience others, and the ways others experience us. We honor that the language we choose to name our experiences matters. As humans, we interpret experiences through language and through the cultural lens of our language. Therefore, people can have different interpretations of the same interaction or life event. We create narratives in our minds to make sense of our life experiences. This is the core of meaning-making. Some of the meaning we make is developed on our own, and some interpretations we've inherited and internalized from others. Narrative therapy helps us consider all of this to help the client rewrite a truer narrative based on their experiences and values. There is no such thing as one objective reality. Ultimately, we each have different realities, even if we have shared experiences.

Using narrative techniques, therapists can help clients identify where core beliefs come from. Once the false belief is identified, therapists can help clients externalize the problem, deconstruct the meaning made of the incident or event, and re-author a truer narrative to facilitate healing, connection, and inner-standing.

Just as books help us understand where our inner struggles come from, narrative therapy encourages us to look at the stories we've picked up along the way and decide if they're really ours to hold. It's like untangling the problems we face from who we are as individuals. The stories we inherit and internalize shape how we see the world and ourselves. By using narrative therapy, we can work through our struggles and find inner peace, while understanding that things aren't always black and white.

One example of how this could look is the following: A client's father abandoned her and Mom when she was a child. The client recorded this memory as Dad leaving because she was unlovable. The therapist works with the client to externalize the problem (abandonment), deconstruct the story (what was going on that might have impacted the parents' relationship), and re-author a truer story to integrate into the client's inner-standing and view (sometimes relationships end, and this has nothing to do with the child).

An important aspect of narrative therapy is the mindset shift from a victim mentality to understanding all the ways we each resist oppression. Even where conflict is present, each of us puts up some kind of fight. Nobody openly receives oppression without resisting in some way. As humans, we are inherently wired to survive and re-sist any harm being done to us. This is a major mindset shift for someone who has been made to believe they've had no agency in life. The entire heart of a narrative-therapy approach is about centering ourselves as the main character of our own lives and owning every-thing that happened before us, around us, and to us. It's about put-ting agency and power back into the hands of the client. It's about helping the most conflict-averse client understand that there is a fighter inside of us all. In therapy, it's like being the hero of your own story. You're not blamed for what happened to you, but you're given the power to change how your story goes from here. It's about real-izing that even if life has been tough, you still have the strength in-side you to keep going and make things better.

Many people start therapy because they are looking for answers. We want to understand why things happen and why they've hap-pened to us. We want help making the larger connections to draw meaning from experiences that are hard to accept. Clients often come to me burdened with the inner conflict that emerges from be-ing cast as a villain in someone else's narrative. Reading offers us the profound gift of self-reflection, helping us discern whether our tur-moil stems from conflict within ourselves, discord with others, or the broader landscape of social issues. Just because you've been cast as a villain doesn't mean you are one—and it doesn't mean you can't change the narrative.

THE CASE OF VICTOR | EMBRACING THE ROLE OF THE VILLAIN FOR SELF-PRESERVATION

Victor, a thirty-five-year-old teacher, sought bibliotherapeutic in-tervention to navigate a complex interpersonal dilemma with a co-teacher he cared about but who often asked him for money and extra time to vent after school—time that he didn't have. He is an empathetic and nurturing friend who often found himself entangled in the lives of colleagues, sometimes at the expense of his mental well-being. At the same time, Victor was caring for his mother, who was undergoing chemotherapy for lung cancer. He was becoming severely depressed at the time we began working together.

Understanding Victor's tendency to prioritize others' needs over his own, we launched into a bibliotherapy journey together. We leaped into literature that explored morally gray characters, protagonists who occupied the nebulous space between hero and villain. One such character we explored was Maddie from Jessica George's novel *Maame*. Maddie is a young woman living in London, navigating the challenges of being the primary caretaker for her father, who has advanced-stage Parkinson's, while also dealing with an overbearing mother who frequently travels to Ghana. Tired of feeling isolated as the only Black person in her workplace, Maddie seizes the opportunity to move out and explore new experiences, including apartment sharing, dating, and pursuing recognition in her career. However, when tragedy strikes, Maddie is forced to confront the complexities of her unconventional family and the importance of finding her place in the world.

Victor and I primarily discussed how Maddie, despite her good intentions and charm, was a character driven by fear and lack of individuation from her mother. Victor began to see parallels between himself and Maddie, as he often bent over backward to help friends and colleagues, sometimes recreating toxic past relationships in the process. He identified with the ways Maddie was overburdened by her responsibilities to others, even when others did not feel responsible for offering reciprocity to her.

Through our conversations, Victor realized the importance of setting boundaries and prioritizing his mental health. We examined the idea that, in some instances, he needed to embrace the role of the villain in others' stories to safeguard his emotional equilibrium.

Exploring a character like Maddie allowed Victor to gain insights into the complexities of human nature and relationships. He came to understand that being the villain in someone else's narrative did not make him a bad person, but rather, a self-preserving individual with healthy boundaries. We also explored how, as the only son of a single mother, his family role reinforced his unconscious tendency to take on responsibilities that were not his.

Victor gradually asserted himself and prioritized his mental health. Although some friends perceived his actions as villainous in their narratives, he found peace in knowing that he was making choices that ultimately improved his life and ability to care for his sick mother from a balanced place. The best part? He stopped self-abandoning and respected himself and his needs more.

Morally gray characters in literature provide valuable lessons, teaching us that sometimes, in the pursuit of self-preservation and well-being, we may need to embrace the role of the villain in someone else's story. In doing so, we assert our boundaries, safeguard our mental health, and embrace a journey toward greater self-empowerment and self-compassion—the same journey Maddie goes on as she learns to prioritize self-love and her own well-being.

In Maddie's words: "And this new Maddie feels great. I mean, really great. She's cool, audacious, and carefree. She's finally everything she's always wanted to be."

BEING THE VILLAIN AND BEING OK WITH IT

As a therapist who incorporates narrative therapy techniques, I'm often asked about the notion of being cast as the villain in someone else's story, which can make many feel ambivalent or upset. My answer is always the same. If you know you have caused someone harm, you should work to repair it. We can only heal what we are aware of. If someone has ostracized you or labeled you a villain, and you have caused harm, then hopefully, it is your objective to do the inner work required to change the circumstances and to repair what you can.

In the inherent complexity of human relationships, it becomes abundantly clear that each of us inevitably assumes the role of the villain in someone else's narrative. Remember, one of the main goals of bibliotherapy is to increase our awareness of interpersonal relationships. This applies to the fact that we cannot please everyone in relationships (especially when we are on a healing journey toward setting healthy boundaries and prioritizing our well-being). This notion, when viewed through the lens of narrative therapy, invites us to explore the multifaceted dimensions of our identities and interactions with others. It is a helpful reminder that the stories we inhabit are interconnected, and our actions, whether intentional or unintentional, can cast us as antagonists in the stories of others.

However, it is essential to recognize that being perceived as a villain does not automatically imply that we have inflicted harm or malice upon another. In fact, it is a stark reminder that our pursuit of self-preservation, our adherence to personal boundaries, and our commitment to our own well-being can occasionally disappoint or clash with the expectations and needs of those around us. This delicate dance between self-care and navigating the emotions of others underscores the complexity of human relationships, offering opportunities for repair when harm has been done. It also offers a deeper understanding of the dynamics that shape our lives, for better or worse.

MORALLY GRAY CHARACTERS AND ASPECTS OF THE SELF

At the core of every narrative arc lies the captivating tension between a protagonist's identity and the challenges they must confront. This narrative nuance is beautifully exemplified by characters who occupy a morally gray territory, which we explored in our earlier discussion of the shadow self.

Life's journey, as we come to realize with time, often demands that we tap into our primal instincts for survival. These instincts can lead us down various paths, from the impulse to flee or freeze to the instinct to appease, connect, or even, metaphorically speaking, "kill." Sometimes, we cast ourselves as villains by abandoning others, ghosting them, or pretending they never existed, mirroring how we fragment our own selves by denying aspects of our humanity. When we avoid acknowledging our rage, envy, lust, greed, or desire for superiority, we perpetuate this self-inflicted division. It is crucial to understand that the fault does not lie in feeling these emotions. As I frequently remind my clients, all feelings are valuable sources of information, revealing the depths of our humanity. The true challenge lies in how we choose to respond to these feelings, consciously and intentionally.

Exploring the experiences and inner lives of morally gray characters in literature, we can find a potent source of healing. In Zora Neale Hurston's classic *Their Eyes Were Watching God*, Tea Cake emerges as a multifaceted character whose actions straddle the line between morality and ambiguity. Initially captivating Janie with his charm and affection, Tea Cake's character gradually reveals a darker side marked by jealousy, impulsiveness, and, ultimately, violence toward Janie. His complex nature challenges conventional notions of morality, prompting readers to question the dynamics of love and power within relationships.

In Gabby Rivera's *Juliet Takes a Breath*, Harlowe Brisbane (a mentor to the titular protagonist, Juliet) stands out as a figure deeply enmeshed in the complexities of activism and personal integrity. Harlowe has progressive ideals but employs controversial methods. Her mentorship often veers into manipulation, forcing Juliet to navigate the challenges that are inherent in the pursuit of social justice.

In Stephen Chbosky's *The Perks of Being a Wallflower*, Patrick embodies the struggle of developing a sense of identity during adolescence as he's torn in different directions by social expectations. Patrick's charismatic persona belies his penchant for risky behavior, including underage drinking and substance abuse. The uncomfortable path to morality and self-discovery unfolds in Patrick's story in disturbingly realistic ways.

These characters, navigating the treacherous territory between right and wrong, resonate with readers because they mirror what it means to be human. Engaging with their stories offers us a profound opportunity to connect with our inner worlds. Morally ambiguous characters challenge the boundaries of conventional morality, prompting us to confront our ethical uncertainties and quandaries— the places where we aren't quite sure what we might do or how we might behave in the face of external pressures and conflicting choices. Bibliotherapy invites us to embrace the spectrum of our moral complexity and the internal conflicts we experience.

Characters' internal conflicts can also offer profound insights into our struggles with self-identity and self-worth, both of which impact how we show up in relationship to others. For marginalized individuals navigating systemic oppression, internal conflict can manifest in various ways, such as grappling with ethical dilemmas, addiction, or decisions that challenge our integrity. We might even go so far as to internalize the ugly narratives that have been created about us by dominant culture—journeying through a maze of mirrors where we find that our reflection is distorted by the perceptions that society has projected onto us. The narratives we engage with in literature encourage us to turn inward, addressing these inner conflicts and seeking a deeper understanding of our authentic selves—who we actually are, not who others imagine us to be.

Literature reveals the truths of the human condition, often demonstrating our tendencies to prioritize preserving relationships at the cost of our own truth. Many of us from marginalized backgrounds have learned the art of silencing our voices or downplaying our truth in the pursuit of maintaining harmony. Literature reminds us that while preserving relationships is admirable, it is essential to discern when such preservation comes at our own expense. Literature increases our awareness of interpersonal relationships by clarifying who we are and how to navigate tensions between our needs and other people's desires for us and from us.

BIBLIOTHERAPEUTIC REFLECTION

One of the ways I like to encourage clients to reconnect with their innate wisdom to self-reflect is letter writing. By expressing ourselves through writing, we deepen our connection to the text and the wisdom it relays to us. In essence, literature becomes more than just stories; it becomes a powerful form of seeing ourselves more clearly and honestly, guiding us on a journey of inner growth and reconnection.

1. For this exercise, pick up a book that you remember reading and enjoying that dealt with a difficult theme(s).
2. Reread the author's opening note for the book (if there isn't one, choose another note from the author in the introduction or elsewhere in the book) and reflect on the approach they took toward preparing the reader for what to expect. What reminders did they provide that felt like care and consideration for you as a reader?
3. After you've done this, write a letter to the author in response to their book. Explain how their words and storytelling impacted you. Describe what you took away from their approach to telling this story. Provide them with any feedback about whatever you felt was missing in their approach. Thank them for the generosity and care they put into writing a story from a trauma-informed lens.

CHAPTER 8

BIBLIOTHERAPY AND NAVIGATING INTERSECTIONALITY
Unveiling The Sociocultural Context In Therapeutic Practice

I believe books are medicine. A library is a medicine cabinet. What can heal one person may not work at all for somebody else. You know when something is healing you, just as you know when something isn't.

—SANDRA CISNEROS, *A House of My Own: Stories from My Life*

As our lives unfold over time, our memories become precious treasures. This experience of growing older provides a unique vantage point, allowing us to gaze back upon our life's journey. We get an opportunity to contemplate the crucial moments that define us. It's similar to gathering the parts of a puzzle: Each piece contributes to the vibrant mosaic of our identity. The pivotal developmental task of becoming an elder lies in making peace with the various trails we've walked and the different aspects of ourselves we've encountered along the way.

Within this chapter, we will explore the profound ways in which literature operates as both a reflection of our life experiences and a conduit to the depth of memory. In the context of intersectionality and culturally relevant bibliotherapy, books act as mirrors, possessing an extraordinary ability to illuminate reflections of different aspects of ourselves and our ever-changing needs and environments.

The narrative power of diverse literature becomes a powerful tool for us to remember ourselves (as individuals and groups), not to mention where we've been and where we're going. The therapeutic power of diverse literature grants us access to both the joyful and painful memories that may reside in the recesses of our minds, freeing us to tell a more complete narrative.

CASE STUDY:
MAYTE

At the beginning of therapy, psychotherapists employ various strategies to engage our clients and establish a strong therapeutic alliance. One fundamental approach is creating a safe and nonjudgmental space where clients feel comfortable expressing themselves, which can be hard to do when a client is referred to therapy by someone else. My client, Mayte, a Dominican elder, was referred to me by her eldest daughter. I wasn't surprised, as most of my Latinx elders are referred to me by family members, and it's often the eldest daughter making the call to set up the intake appointment. The first time I met with Mayte, she arrived at the clinic with her eldest daughter and two younger daughters.

Throughout the entire intake, I noticed that her daughters would speak for her, even when I offered to facilitate the session in Spanish so that Mayte would understand. Mayte had suffered a traumatic brain injury and, as a result, lost much of her memory. The family reported that doctors were hopeful her memories would return, but there was no way of predicting when this would happen. I sat and listened attentively while taking mental notes. I noted that every time Mayte tried to speak, she took long pauses and turned red in the face, growing frustrated with herself for being unable to articulate her many thoughts and feelings. I was patient and encouraged her to take all the time she needed. In between gently redirecting her daughters to let her finish her sentences, I would reinforce how much love I could feel in the room. I was looking forward to my first solo session with Mayte and curious about how much of herself she might allow to emerge in the room alone with me.

My goal for the first session was simply to demonstrate active listening, empathy, support, and genuine interest in Mayte's experience. I wanted her to feel heard, validated, and understood. The first session with Mayte flowed seamlessly. I could tell she was excited to have a space for herself to be with a caring professional who wasn't focused on putting her through exercises or judging her improvement or lack thereof.

The first thing she noticed in my office was a copy of Sandra Cisneros' *The House on Mango Street* on my bookshelf. She placed her hand on the edge of the sofa and attempted to lift herself to her feet. Her cane was far out of reach near the door, and I could see she was struggling. I got up right away and asked her if I could help reach whatever she was grasping for. She immediately said, "Tienes mi libro favorito!" *You have my favorite book!* I grabbed it from the shelf, and she eagerly reached for it. I shared that this is one of my favorites, too.

She began to talk for the next forty minutes or so about how much the book reminded her of her grandfather. I asked if there was any chapter or scene that brought back those positive feelings, and she said yes, the section titled "Papa Who Wakes Up Tired in the Dark":

Your *abuelito* is dead, Papa says early one morning in my room. *Está muerto,* and then as if he just heard the news himself, crumples like a coat and cries, my brave Papa cries. I have never seen my Papa cry and don't know what to do.

I know he will have to go away, that he will take a plane to Mexico, all the uncles and aunts will be there, and they will have a black-and-white photo taken in front of the tomb with flowers shaped like spears in a white vase because this is how they send the dead away in that country.

Because I am the oldest, my father has told me first, and now it is my turn to tell the others. I will have to explain why we can't play. I will have to tell them to be quiet today.

My Papa, his thick hands and thick shoes, who wakes up tired in the dark, who combs his hair with water, drinks his coffee, and is gone before we wake, today is sitting on my bed.

And I think if my own Papa died what would I do. I hold my Papa in my arms. I hold and hold and hold him.

Mayte asked me to read it again, aloud to her. I asked if she'd like me to read it in English or Spanish. I had both copies available in my office. Her eyes lit up with expectancy as she asked me to read in Spanish. When I did, she closed her eyes to really soak in the words and let them wash over her. I could see tears form at the edge of her right eye, and I controlled my impulse to reach over and grab the tissue box. Instead, I kept reading. When I was done, she let out a deep breath and released her tears. I sat as a witness to her relief, and it was a moment's notice before I saw the drops land on my necklace and realized I was crying, too.

"Pedrito," she said. I asked her who Pedrito was, and she said it was the name of her father. In all the time she struggled to remember her own name and that of her daughters, connecting through literature helped her access her father's memory—so much so that she remembered his name.

BIBLIOTHERAPY IN PRACTICE:
IN THE AFTERMATH OF A TRAUMATIC BRAIN INJURY

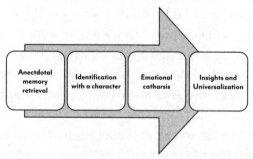

Anecdotal memory retrieval: My client reads "Papa Who Wakes up Tired in the Dark" and remembers her late grandfather.

Identification with a character: She relates to Papa's grief. She quotes "…crumples like a coat and cries, my brave Papa cries."

Emotional catharsis: My client expresses anger and frustration at all the things she cannot remember.

Insight and universalization: My client remembers the burdens placed on her as the eldest daughter and feels less alone in her recovery struggle while remembering that others have recovered from a TBI in the past.

In a 2015 interview with *Electric Literature*, Sandra Cisneros is quoted as saying: "I don't believe in best books because I firmly believe books are medicine. What heals me might not work for you."

This is exactly how I feel about bibliotherapy and one of the reasons why, as a clinician, I don't make general book lists, which I'm often asked to make as wide-ranging prescriptions for depression, anxiety, etc. I believe in pairing readers with the literature they need in the moment they come to my practice. If books are medicine, everyone's prescription needs to be tailor-made. Every dosage needs to be measured and considered with respect to the chemistry of one's body, needs, and history. And, if books are medicine, who has the right to ban them?

The House on Mango Street was banned after an angry Texan mother requested that the book be removed from library shelves. She made claims about the narrative that simply weren't true, and her efforts were rewarded. The book was banned. I read Cisneros's response to this mother and was deeply touched by her words and the way she extended tenderness in the face of deep hostility. Cisneros responded, "May you find the right books to fall in love with and be transformed by, and may those books that don't meet your needs be placed gently back on the bookshelf. I wish you well in your journey of self-discovery." She did not clap back or get defensive. She did not take it personally that this woman could not honor her story and truly missed the point of her telling it. She simply wished the woman well on her path. Not everyone will relate to our intersectional experiences. Cisneros' response is a master class in self-care and boundaries for all writers!

Mayte's story vividly illustrates the importance of understanding a client's intersectionality and emphasizes the need for therapists to recognize and understand our clients' unique sociocultural context. Kimberlé Williams Crenshaw, a critical race theory thought leader and American civil rights activist, was the first scholar to introduce the concept of intersectionality. Intersectionality is understood as "the complex, cumulative way in which the effects of multiple forms of discrimination combine, overlap, or intersect, especially in the experiences of marginalized individuals or groups." Intersectionality provides a way to understand how the many different aspects of our identities frame our experiences in the world. While oppression exists on many different levels, we are all impacted differently based on the ever-changing landscape of what's happening around us and the systems we interact with in our daily lives.

As Mayte grappled with her recovery journey, her Latinx identity and family dynamics played a significant role in shaping her coming to therapy. Being referred by her eldest daughter highlighted the familial bonds deeply ingrained in Latinx communities and value systems, where the role of family is paramount. The language barrier Mayte faced, with her daughters speaking on her behalf, reflects the complexities that arise in the therapy room, especially when cultural nuances intersect with cognitive challenges.

Understanding intersectionality in therapy involves acknowledging the layered impact of identities and experiences on an individual's mental health. For Mayte, being a Latinx woman, a mother, and someone recovering from a traumatic brain injury intersected in important ways, influencing the support she would respond to in the therapy room. Therapists must navigate these intersections with sensitivity to promote a healing environment that respects cultural nuances, language preferences, and family dynamics.

Mayte's connection to the work of Sandra Cisneros further underlines the multifaceted nature of her identity. The resonance she felt with *The House on Mango Street,* which triggered memories of her father, reflects the power of shared cultural narratives in therapeutic exploration. The moment where literature served as a bridge to Mayte's memories emphasizes the importance of cultural competence in therapy. This example highlights how therapists can leverage shared cultural references to deepen the therapeutic alliance, creating a space where clients feel validated. Equipped with an understanding of intersectionality, therapists can navigate clinical complexities effectively, ultimately contributing to more holistic and culturally sensitive mental health care.

By acknowledging and honoring the multiple aspects of a person's identity, such as race, gender, sexuality, and socioeconomic status, we create a space where clients feel seen, valued, and understood. This inclusive approach allows for more authentic and effective therapeutic relationships, where clients can explore their experiences with greater depth and authenticity, ultimately promoting healing and growth.

FOSTERING PSYCHOLOGICAL WELL-BEING THROUGH INCLUSIVE THERAPY

In mental health care, there is often a prevailing misconception that psychological well-being is solely an individual concern. This narrow perspective fails to acknowledge the significant role that psychosocial support, or the lack thereof, plays in the mental health of individuals within marginalized communities.

The truth is that many marginalized communities face systemic barriers to accessing adequate mental health resources, from socioeconomic disparities to cultural stigmatization. To bridge this gap, we must shift our focus from viewing mental health as an isolated issue to recognizing it as inherently linked to the socio-environmental factors that shape our lives. Achieving this broader perspective requires community-based interventions and psychosocial support systems that can empower individuals within marginalized communities to navigate unique challenges using the tools that work for them and have historically been employed in our communities. One of those approaches involves storytelling and connecting to stories.

Bibliotherapy, with its holistic approach to healing, offers a distinctive pathway toward addressing disparities in accessing mental health resources. By providing literature that reflects the experiences, struggles, and triumphs of marginalized individuals, bibliotherapy serves as a bridge to psychosocial support. It helps readers see themselves in the narratives, fostering a sense of belonging and validation that is often missing in traditional mental health care settings. By offering a diverse array of books that resonate with the lived experiences of marginalized communities, bibliotherapy uniquely contributes to expanding the psychosocial support network, ultimately promoting mental well-being and resilience in underserved populations. If you've never thought of your book collection as a psychosocial support, I'm here to tell you that it most definitely is!

Consider the impact of personal libraries and access to books on readers' psychosocial well-being and mental health. I immediately think of programs that hire "balm readers," who read to patients undergoing chemotherapy in hospitals. These initiatives, even in settings as diverse as hospitals, highlight the therapeutic power of literature. Whether reading privately, being read to, or engaging in shared reading experiences, the act of connecting through literature feels like a form of medicine, especially during times of illness or distress. For many, being read to evokes positive childhood memories of nurturing caregivers who nourished them through storytelling. For others who may not have had this experience growing up, access to literature offers a new opportunity for nurturing and connection. Books serve as a form of medicine, offering both literal and figurative healing to readers, providing comfort, solace, and a sense of connection in times of need.

Libraries as Centers of Healing

If books are medicine, then libraries are pharmacies where we can go to pick up our prescriptions at no cost. Libraries are the main providers of the medicine that's most easily accessible in our communities. When libraries were made public, the medicine that books provide became available to the most invisible among us.

Libraries are one of the most pivotal communal spaces in our society. In her book *The Library Book*, Susan Orlean writes:

> The publicness of the public library is an increasingly rare commodity. It becomes harder all the time to think of places that welcome everyone and don't charge any money for the warm embrace. The commitment to inclusion is so powerful that many decisions about the library hinge on whether or not a particular choice would cause a subset of the public to feel uninvited.

Libraries are for everyone and make literature accessible to those who might struggle to access books without their presence. As we briefly explored in Chapter 2, the creation of public libraries has played a significant role in community mental health care.

Public libraries significantly contribute to mental well-being by offering various resources and programs. Libraries serve as valuable hubs of information on mental health, providing a range of books, articles, and resources for self-healing practice, self-help guides, and psychoeducational materials on mental health conditions. This access to information empowers people to educate themselves, which fosters a deeper understanding of what mental health challenges can look like, reducing stigma and encouraging individuals to seek out support. Public libraries actively contribute to reducing the stigma associated with mental health. By providing judgment-free spaces for accessing mental health resources, libraries normalize discussions around well-being, creating a more inclusive and understanding community for people who may not experience that support within their families of origin. They also prioritize inclusivity by offering accommodations for diverse needs and creating safe spaces for individuals of all backgrounds and abilities.

Libraries host community programs and events that promote mental health and well-being, including workshops, support groups, and presentations on a range of topics. These events facilitate community engagement, provide learning opportunities, and connect people with valuable resources and services, contributing to a collective sense of belonging and support within communities at large. Acting as community hubs, libraries foster social connections and combat feelings of isolation. Through activities like book clubs and discussion groups, people can connect with others who share similar interests or experiences, also enhancing their sense of belonging and social supports.

Some public libraries incorporate bibliotherapy programs, where trained librarians recommend books and reading materials as therapeutic tools to support mental health. This approach recognizes the therapeutic benefits of reading fiction or self-help books in providing comfort, inspiration, and insights that contribute to personal growth and self-reflection practice. Not everyone can afford to curate a personal library. The library offers those individuals a chance to engage with literature free of charge.

THE MAIN PILLARS OF MENTAL HEALTH

Understanding mental health involves recognizing the interconnectedness of emotional, psychological, and social well-being. These pillars are deeply entwined in our fast-paced, capitalist society. In addition, we must consider factors like financial, physical, and spiritual well-being, as they collectively shape our overall wellness. It is essential to view these aspects from an individual perspective and through the lens of communal mental health. In Western culture, these pillars often appear separate, but in reality, they are intricately linked.

As a young social worker, my training emphasized the significance of evaluating mental health by observing changes in baseline functioning. Baseline functioning encompasses a person's typical cognitive, emotional, social, and behavioral abilities under usual circumstances. It serves as a reference point for clinicians to assess shifts over time, highlighting the interconnectedness of individual and communal well-being.

The concept of baseline functioning becomes crucial when determining whether symptoms are within the usual range. Unfortunately, prevailing models sometimes suggest enduring pain before seeking support, which reinforces an individualist mentality. The issue with this is that many people lack a safety net and real social supports. An individualist mentality forces people to maintain a façade of well-being. The pressure to appear functional in a capitalist society leads to concealing struggles, creating a societal disconnect. Recognizing our interconnectedness allows us to shift toward a more communal understanding of mental health, where collective well-being supports individual flourishing.

Through our involvement in book communities, book clubs, book events, and book retreats, we can find like-minded people to befriend on our journey. The only way to heal our relational wounds is to enter back into community with one another in a way that allows our full humanity to be present and witnessed. In *How We Show Up: Reclaiming Family, Friendship, and Community*, Mia Birdsong writes:

That level of smart, open, thoughtful communication requires a willingness to be vulnerable that doesn't come easy to everyone. You're creating a relationship, which is not transactional. You're creating connection and intimacy. I think that's why some people try to keep distance- intimacy. What's made my relationships with nonblood family good and juicy and useful, and just giving me life, is that they're intimate. At the core of it is that I can be vulnerable, and put all my shit out there, and not be judged for it, and have it held. That's explicitly understood.

Birdsong beautifully captures the essence of building intimate and meaningful relationships within our communities. These words underscore the importance of vulnerability and open communication in creating genuine connections that enrich our lives. However, in a society that often prioritizes individualism and self-sufficiency, the value of community support for mental health can be overlooked. The truth is, we are social beings wired for connection, and our mental well-being thrives when we have a network of supportive relationships. Building community allows us to share our vulnerabilities, fears, and struggles without fear of judgment, knowing we will be met with understanding and empathy. In contrast, an individualist mindset that emphasizes self-reliance can isolate us and hinder our ability to seek help or support when we need it most. By embracing the idea that we need each other, we cultivate stronger bonds within our communities and create a nurturing environment where our mental health can flourish.

Community mental health supports our emotional, psychological, and social well-being because it provides access to people and programs that help us be in relationship to others. There is no better example of this than the public library, where historically the homeless, the mentally ill, the poor family, and the person in need have been able to access literature, classes, book clubs, community support, and more.

THE PANDEMIC THAT REMINDED US OF
THE IMPORTANCE OF COMMUNITY

The COVID-19 pandemic and its continued aftermath have had a significant impact on mental health in our society. Isolation, grief, economic stress, and uncertainties during the pandemic have contributed to increased rates of anxiety, depression, and other mental health issues. The pandemic exacerbated a multitude of preexisting stressors, such as medical and mental health concerns, social isolation, economic challenges, and disruptions in daily routines, all while contributing significantly to increased uncertainty. These factors, combined with preexisting risk factors that impact some communities more than others, have contributed to the mental health crisis we currently find ourselves in. The Centers for Disease Control and Prevention (CDC) has recognized the mental health implications of the pandemic and highlighted several factors contributing to the crisis:

- *Increased Stress*: The pandemic has caused widespread stress and anxiety due to concerns about personal health, the health of loved ones, job insecurity, financial pressures, and the overall uncertainty surrounding the future.

- *Economic Factors*: Economic downturns or disparities can lead to job losses, financial struggles, and reduced access to mental health services, which can exacerbate stress and mental health problems.

- *Social Media and Technology*: The rise of social media and increased use of technology can negatively affect mental health. Cyberbullying, online harassment, and excessive use of social media have been associated with increased rates of anxiety and depression, especially among younger populations.

- *Climate Change and Natural Disasters*: The effects of climate change, such as extreme weather events, natural disasters, and displacement, can lead to trauma and psychological distress.

- *Access to Mental Health Services*: Limited access to affordable and quality mental health services can be a significant barrier for people seeking help.

- *Grief and Loss*: Many individuals have experienced the loss of loved ones, as well as other losses, such as jobs, income, and social connections. The grieving process and the associated emotional challenges can contribute to mental health difficulties.

- *Limited Access to Mental Health Services*: The pandemic has strained mental health resources and limited access to in-person mental health care. This has made it challenging for individuals to seek help and receive necessary support.

The mental health crisis in the United States is a complex issue influenced by various social, economic, and systemic factors. Efforts to address the crisis involve improving access to mental health services, reducing stigma, promoting mental health education and awareness, and implementing policies that prioritize mental well-being.

In our current challenging environment, therapeutic approaches like bibliotherapy offer valuable tools for coping, self-expression, and building a sense of community. For those who adore literature, there's an innate understanding of how our love for books serves as a source of respite from the daily grind, whether we consciously recognize the psychological connections or not. The significance lies not solely in being evidence-based but in the emotional impact our books have on us. They provide a space for us to be present, to escape, to slow down, to laugh, to cry, or even to express frustration by chucking a book across the room. This love for literature becomes a self-paced journey through various emotional states, emphasizing the idea that feeling precedes being.

It's important to mention that research supports the mental health benefits of reading, particularly during challenging times like the COVID-19 lockdown in 2020. Studies indicate that individuals who engaged in more reading experienced fewer mental health issues, including depression, anxiety, and stress. As we navigated confinement, embracing rewarding hobbies like reading was recommended for leisure and psychological well-being, as well as improved sleep, enhanced imagination, cognitive exercise, knowledge expansion, literacy, and overall quality of life. This reinforces the idea that our love for literature actively contributes to supporting our mental health in diverse and meaningful ways.

When it's hard to find the words, books help us access language. When it's hard to identify our thoughts and emotions, we can find comfort between the covers of a good book. We can find inner clarity there, too. My clients are already reading, and by asking them to bring their literature into the therapy room, I am better able to understand their desires. Incorporating the literature my clients are reading into therapy also provides a way for me to assess the full scope of their hopelessness. I can use literature as a lifeguard to prevent hopelessness from drowning them completely.

Feeling like all hope is lost is a common reaction in life, especially when the world keeps moving forward, expecting us to keep up. There's this pressure to keep going, even when we're struggling to keep our balance and feeling overwhelmed by life's challenges. Many people are facing difficult situations, like kids going to school hungry or experiencing abuse at home, and families breaking apart under the strain of isolation and lack of support. While things might not always be as dire as they seem, it's easy to slip into all-or-nothing thinking, especially when you're living through tough times with no end in sight. When life keeps knocking you down, it's natural to feel like giving up. I think it's important to talk more openly about that feeling of hopelessness, to acknowledge how overwhelming it can be when there's no relief in sight. We need to recognize the power of connections with others in keeping hope alive and giving us the belief that things can improve.

From my experience, I've found solace and healing in places like libraries, book communities, and friendships centered around books. These spaces provide a much-needed pause and a glimmer of hope in difficult times.

BIBLIOTHERAPEUTIC REFLECTION:

Let's reflect on the intertwined themes of intersectionality, banned books, and justice in the realm of mental health. Consider the following questions and prompts to deepen your engagement with these concepts:

1. *Intersectionality in the Therapy Room*: Reflect on your identity and the ways in which various aspects, such as culture, ethnicity, gender, and family dynamics, intersect to shape your experiences and perceptions. How might these intersections influence your approach to seeking or providing mental health support?

2. *Banned Books and Self-Discovery*: Explore the idea of banned books as catalysts for self-discovery. Have you ever encountered a book that challenged your perspectives or made you question societal norms? How did this experience contribute to your personal growth and understanding of justice?

3. *Justice and Collective Mental Health*: Consider the concept of justice as a factor in social and collective mental health. How do societal injustices impact mental well-being on a broader scale? In what ways can therapeutic spaces contribute to social justice, and how might literature play a role in fostering awareness and change?

4. *Cultural Competence in Therapy*: Building on Mayte's story, reflect on the importance of cultural competence in therapy. How can therapists create inclusive spaces that honor diverse identities and experiences? Share your thoughts on the role of shared cultural narratives in therapeutic exploration.

Feel free to explore these questions personally or engage in discussions with peers, book clubs, or therapy groups. Remember, the journey of self-discovery and healing is unique to everyone, and literature often serves as a guiding light in navigating the complexities of our collective human experience.

CHAPTER 9

BIBLIOTHERAPY THROUGH THE PHASES OF LIFE

I believe that my time was a remarkable one. I am aware that we are now living in a world overrun by cruelty and destruction, and as our earth disintegrates and our spirits numb, we lose moral purpose and creative vision. But still I must believe, as I always have, that our best times lie ahead, and that in the final analysis, along the way we shall be comforted by one another. That is my song.

—HARRY BELAFONTE, *My Song: A Memoir*

What captivates me most about literature is its ability to guide us through the unique demands of each life phase. Growing older brings wisdom that is often undervalued in our society, especially beyond fifty. Books serve as mirrors reflecting the truth about our emotional needs throughout our lives—at every age and stage. Many of my retired clients find contentment in reading; some even volunteer as "balm readers" for cancer patients undergoing chemotherapy. From childhood's formative years to the twists of adolescence and the complexities of adulthood, literature provides an invaluable opportunity to access self-knowledge in our golden years.

Ancestor Harry Belafonte's words, shared in the context of his experiences, resonate with the multilayered experiences that shape our lives. He reminds us of our place in an ever-changing world marred by cruelty, emphasizing that the remedy lies in communal connection and the relationships we forge with ourselves and with one another. Facing the challenges of growing older, Belafonte's steadfast belief in a brighter future inspires us to evolve continually. There is no end point to our unfolding. Adulthood, in essence, is about navigating bodily changes, shifting roles, and various life experiences. Refusing to honor these changes traps us emotionally, hindering our growth.

Erik Erikson's psychosocial stages theory is a useful framework for therapists in understanding human development across the lifespan, revealing the unique challenges each stage presents for self-realization. Before I worked directly with adults and elders at Literapy NYC, my career began as a middle school social worker, supporting young people and their families. I've been able to incorporate the use of literature with clients of all ages and have found that books enhance therapeutic progress no matter who the intervention is built for.

In my fourteen years as a school social worker, I cherished the opportunity to serve vulnerable youth who struggled to access mental health services outside of school. I found that incorporating reflections about life into the books we read in the ELA classroom became a great tool to get students reflecting on their developing values and identities.

Bridging theory and practice, we will uncover the profound impact of bibliotherapy on people throughout their life phases, and I will show you how I helped those young people link their insights to a deeper understanding of their parents' immigrant experiences. This exploration showcases the central role literature plays in fostering connections, understanding emotional needs, and building bridges between generations in an increasingly complex world.

CASE STUDY:
ESPERANZA RISING BY PAM MUÑOZ RYAN

Using the understanding of human development that Erikson suggests, I've often referred to Erikson's fifth stage, known as Identity versus Role Confusion, when working with adolescents. During this stage, typically occurring in the teenage years (around twelve to eighteen years old), we face the challenge of forming a strong and coherent sense of identity or experiencing confusion about who we are and what we want to become. Erikson believed that successfully resolving this identity crisis for teenagers would lead to the development of a well-defined and stable sense of self. This includes understanding one's values, beliefs, aspirations, and life goals. Additionally, a positive resolution of this stage enables youth to make meaningful connections to roles and relationships that align with their identity as first-generation American students navigating the divide between cultures—a divide that often leaves children from immigrant families feeling disconnected and disjointed.

In the words of Jennifer Mullan, author of *Decolonizing Therapy*: "We are not broken beyond repair; we are awaiting to be reminded that we can return Home. Acknowledging the embodied legacy of oppression and colonization is not at odds with healing, but is an essential step on the journey toward healing."

One example of bibliotherapy with teens in the classroom environment that I will never forget was reading *Esperanza Rising*, by Pam Muñoz Ryan, with eighth-grade students during summer school. My class was a group of all Black and Latinx girls. All NYC kids, they came from different walks of life but were all first-generation children of immigrants. One student was being raised by her grandmother, an immigrant from the Dominican Republic; another was mourning the loss of her father and struggling to understand the inevitability of mortality; and the other two girls were stepsisters being raised by a single mother, an immigrant from Mexico.

I was excited to read the book with these students because it tells the story of a Mexican family forced to flee their home country after Esperanza's father dies and her family finds themselves in a dangerous situation. It included a lot of themes that address the many transitions we experience in life from the lens of a young Latinx girl who immigrates to the States. When the family comes to the U.S., the quality of their lives drastically decreases.

Esperanza is the kind of narrator you trust to tell the truth about how difficult it can be to adjust when life suddenly takes you down an unexpected pivot—a trauma-informed middle-grade read of the best kind! Better yet, Esperanza reflected the age and cultural background of the students in my classroom. Each student in this class related to Esperanza and was invested in her story, which I knew would make for a meaningful discussion around what my students valued. I looked forward to seeing what conversations the story would bring up for the girls. My goal in reading this book with them was to support the goal of shaping and strengthening their sense of self.

One day in class, we were reading aloud a scene in which Esperanza's mother falls ill due to an infection spreading through her body and the exhaustion caused by her physical labor to make ends meet. Christmas is approaching, and it's abundantly clear that Esperanza will not enjoy the holiday as she used to when her father was alive and could shower her with all the material gifts she could dream of. When Esperanza's friend Isabel asks what she wants for Christmas, Esperanza tells Isabel she only wishes for her mother to get well and for more work so she can help her mother out financially. When Esperanza asks Isabel what she wants, she responds, "That's easy. I want anything!"

Isabel's answer surprises Esperanza, who is yearning for the days of the past. As Esperanza cries herself to sleep, Isabel overhears and asks to sleep in her bed. With her, she brings a collection of small dolls made of yarn that she arranges in between them, under the covers. The next line seemed to resonate deeply with my students that day: "Esperanza stared into the dark. Isabel had nothing, but she also had everything. Esperanza wanted what she had. She wanted so few worries that something as simple as a yarn doll would make her happy."

"What does she mean by she had nothing, but she had everything?" one student asked.

"I think it's saying that she had everything because she was happy enough with her yarn dolls," another student responded.

"Yeah, Esperanza wants to be happy enough, but she can't be because Mami is sick, and she has a lot of other worries on her mind," said another girl.

This exchange led to a full-classroom discussion about the idea of contentment and what it feels like to be content. The girls were all very bothered that Esperanza was so discontent. They wanted her suffering to be relieved immediately and did not want the school day to end before we read the next chapter.

The students were preoccupied with the question of whether Esperanza's mother would die like her father did. Would she be left alone in the world? Of the four, most of them could not handle the idea of that. Some could relate to the frustration of having so many questions and feelings but not enough answers. Many had seen their parents and grandparents push their bodies so hard doing physical labor that there was no room left for processing emotions at the end of a long, exhausting day.

The students found comfort in the moments when Esperanza could speak honestly with her mother and hear her mother's earnest responses. They craved more connection with their own exhausted parents. This made me reflect on the utility of language, how we are often unable to be seen, felt, and understood in relationship to one another when we cannot access the words. The next day in class, the students were happy to share stories of processing Esperanza's narrative with their immigrant parents. They, too, valued their parents. They wanted to make it known.

BIBLIOTHERAPY IN PRACTICE:

TEEN FOCUS: IDENTITY OR CONFUSION?

Personal Values	➡	What matters to me?
Beliefs	➡	What do I believe?
Goals	➡	What do I want?
Sense of Self	➡	Who am I and who do I want to be?

"Esperanza stared into the dark. Isabel had nothing, but she also had everything. Esperanza wanted what she had. She wanted so few worries that something as simple as a yarn doll would make her happy."

GROUP BIBLIOTHERAPY WITH PARENTS

One of my favorite aspects of being a school social worker is curating and facilitating parent workshops. This has proven to be an effective way to provide parents with support and resources and to build a bridge between school and the home. After reading *Esperanza Rising* with the students, I decided to host a book talk with parents about the text. While planning the parent workshop, I decided to take a group bibliotherapy approach and pulled some excerpts from an adult memoir that would help parents make meaningful connections to their lived experiences as immigrants.

I invited parents to join me in reading *Enrique's Journey* by Sonia Nazario. We explored the powerful story of a seventeen-year-old boy's quest to reunite with his mother in the United States. This shared experience became a bridge for parents to connect with their stories and the lasting impact of generational challenges.

As we read together, parents discovered new language to express long-buried memories and emotions. This collective reading deepened their self-understanding and equipped them to unabashedly discuss the complexities of immigration with their kids; many of them had never had that conversation before. By navigating the developmental task of their own life stage, Intimacy versus Isolation (Erikson's sixth stage), parents could separate their emotional needs from their role as caregivers. This nurtured stronger family bonds. This process highlighted how opening up is crucial for connection. It also illuminated how many caregivers are parenting who have never actively been parented with emotional intimacy at the forefront. Providing this group of parents with this experience of group bibliotherapy and parent coaching became a meaningful tool to bridge those gaps.

The shared exploration of Enrique's challenges provided a safe space for parents to reflect on their immigration stories, including their sacrifices and struggles. Through group discussions and reflective exercises, parents unearthed long-buried memories and emotions, finding new ways to articulate their experiences and engage with their children about the complexities of immigration. Below are some of those ways.

Sharing Personal Reflections: During group discussions, parents were encouraged to share their personal reflections on key moments in *Enrique's Journey* that resonated with their experiences. For example, they discussed how Enrique's longing for family reminded them of their own feelings of separation from loved ones during their immigration journey. Reflective questions such as "What emotions does this scene evoke for you?" and "How does Enrique's story relate to your own journey?" prompted parents to explore their thoughts and feelings in a supportive group setting.

Mapping Emotional Journeys: Another reflective exercise involved creating emotional journey maps inspired by Enrique's experiences. Parents were given blank timelines and asked to mark significant events in Enrique's life, along with their emotional responses to these events. This activity allowed parents to visually map out their emotional journeys alongside Enrique's, identifying common themes and connections between their experiences and those depicted in the book.

Role-Playing and Perspective-Taking: Group discussions also included role-playing exercises in which parents were asked to take on the perspectives of different characters in *Enrique's Journey*. For instance, they role-played as Enrique's mother, imagining her feelings of guilt and longing as she grappled with the decision to leave her son behind. By stepping into the shoes of these characters, parents gained a deeper understanding of the complexities of family separation and immigration, fostering compassion for both the characters in the book and for themselves. This collective reading experience deepened their self-awareness and equipped them with valuable insights and language to navigate conversations with their kids about their shared heritage and family history. By engaging with their own developmental tasks of intimacy versus isolation, parents were able to cultivate stronger bonds within their families, enhancing a sense of connection with their children and promoting intergenerational understanding. This process underscored the importance of emotional openness and vulnerability in nurturing healthy family relationships and provided parents with a transformative tool for bridging generational gaps and fostering intergenerational dialogue.

NURTURING STABILITY: CULTIVATING NERVOUS-SYSTEM REGULATION IN UNPARENTED YOUTH

When I was young, my therapist was the first person who taught me what a healthy connection based on reciprocity felt like. It took a long time for her to earn my trust due to my abandonment issues and childhood wounds. She once told me to take the boxing gloves off. Some people are fighters (the fight instinct), some people are people pleasers (the fawn instinct), some people are runners (the flight instinct), and some people freeze (the freeze instinct). I always put up a fight. Historically, this is what helped me stay alive—not just physically but mentally and emotionally, too.

What would it be like not to fight? It's a question I seek the answer to until this very day. It's a question that I became even more passionate about answering once I became a social worker in the Bronx. As a result, I've found a way to help my clients do what I've managed to accomplish for myself: learn to seek and find their own answers in stories that hold space for them and their unique experiences.

In my counseling office, where the struggles of students often go unseen by the systems in place, I encountered the profound impact of systemic challenges, particularly in the life of my student David. David, the son of an incarcerated mother battling drug addiction, had faced an uphill battle since early childhood. The education system, not designed to address mental health risk factors in our children, further complicates the journey for Black and Brown youth like David.

Navigating oppressive systems forces these young people, like David, to become adept fighters. Some adopt an aggressive approach, actively pursuing their needs, while others move cautiously, waiting for the opportune moment to respond. Understanding this nuanced dynamic is crucial for anyone attempting to build trust with a youth like David. Trust, in this context, is not a passive concept but an active exercise that requires intentional steps to demonstrate that you are not a threat.

As a therapist, entering the life of a young person without a safety net, like David, involves dismantling the pervasive influence of power. The question looming in their minds is whether you are a part of the system that threatens to render them invisible or if you are someone capable of helping them survive it. This evaluation extends further to determine if you are an asset or merely another entity they must guard against. In an environment where threats can arise from anyone at any time, building trust becomes a complex and essential foundational aspect of therapeutic intervention.

My life experiences uniquely equipped me to guide students like David toward finding ease in their nervous systems. Mariel Buqué, author of *Break the Cycle*, writes about clients who never experienced attunement from their caregivers. She explores how clinicians can provide our clients with a reparative experience by offering and establishing security in the relationship we build with them, based on helping these clients experience balance, consistency, and care in the therapeutic relationship. My school counseling office, free from the need for constant vigilance and the metaphorical boxing gloves, became a sanctuary where David could embrace vulnerability and initiate his healing, at least during his time at school and within my care.

CASE STUDY:
DAVID

David is a student I will never forget. Few people would call him sweet, but I will name him that. He was scrawny, but mostly because he was malnourished—a skinny boy in the fifth grade with a reputation for being unpredictable. He liked arson, picked at his skin, and would lie to an adult in authority without flinching. Teachers were afraid of him, and administrators were constantly on edge about whether his behavioral episodes would cause the network any liability. People just told me they gave up on working with him and genuinely felt like there was nothing more they could do. In this case example, my boxing gloves came in handy.

I learned that David had been surrounded by distress and anguish his entire life. Born in prison to an incarcerated mother who would become addicted to drugs after reuniting with him, he was never provided with any consistency. Here was a kid who was always on edge and in trouble. No matter what he did, he just couldn't seem to follow the rules, stay in line, remain in his seat, and listen to the adult in the room who was speaking. Whatever he had to do, he would escape the situation. I decided I wouldn't let him escape me.

When I first met David, I engaged him in the classroom but paid him little attention. I focused on helping the other students, supporting the teacher with tasks, and tightening up the routines in the flow of the day. I could feel David observing my every word and interaction. That's exactly what I wanted him to do.

When we moved to working in small groups, I worked in the group adjacent to David's, in close enough proximity to interact with him, too—close enough to pick up a pencil that had fallen from his desk or answer a reading question. Months passed, and I knew David had let down his guard enough to consider that I was not at all a threat to him. When I found him with the dean in the hallway one day, I could tell the dean was exhausted. David had climbed on top of the radiator and refused to come down.

"I'm a grown man, and I'm not going to pick him up from there or put my hands on a kid," the dean said.

I understood, and I was happy to help if he'd allow me to. I could see the relief on his face when I said it. He went back to his office and asked that I walk David over when we were done talking. I was grateful that the dean trusted me, but more so, grateful for a moment alone with David. This would be a true test of whether I had earned a modicum of his trust or not.

"I'm going to jump," David said.

"What?" I asked.

"I'm going to jump down," he repeated and placed his foot over the ledge of the windowsill he'd climbed onto over the radiator when the dean and I weren't looking.

"OK, jump, but if you break your legs, that's not on me," I said.

"You would get in trouble," he said with a sly grin.

"I've gotten into trouble before," I said, "but you getting hurt still wouldn't be my fault."

"You don't care about getting into trouble?" he asked.

"Not if I know I did nothing wrong," I said.

He slowly climbed down from the radiator and met me safely on the ground. The dean had walked back to our side of the hallway and looked at me, clearly impressed when he saw David on the ground and off the unit. I smiled back, though I didn't feel very impressed. The entire time, I didn't think David wanted to jump or climb the radiator. Instead, I think he was trying to gain control of the situation. His behaviors were all externalized: lighting things on fire, running, hiding, climbing, screaming. He had to learn to take the boxing gloves off.

When David would come with me into the counseling room, all he wanted to do was read. When I observed him in the classroom, I noticed that SSR (silent, sustained reading) was the only time he remained seated. He enjoyed stories, I quickly realized. When I asked him about his favorite books, he told me about *The Snowy Day* by Ezra Jack Keats and *Corduroy* by Don Freeman, so I read those aloud to him. In my counseling office, I had a cozy reading nook with a plush carpet and several bean bags lined up along the wall. During these sessions in my office, David was more regulated than usual. It was the only time I didn't hear him make a sound. It was the only time his body was at ease.

Reading to David and witnessing the difference it made for him fostered my love of bibliotherapy and the therapeutic power of reading. The power of storytelling helps us transcend our present circumstances, no matter what is happening around us or inside of us. I knew this personally as much as I was learning it professionally. Before this student encounter, it hadn't occurred to me to use books in the counseling room with kids in this way. When working with or teaching children, one focus of integrating literature is to teach social/emotional skills. The students were already reading for their social/emotional learning in the classroom, but this felt sense of connection and emotional safety in my office was something unique.

David taught me that books and stories are so much more than academic learning tools or ways to teach moral character. Reading the stories of others, whether fictional or true, fosters understanding and connection and provides a useful, accessible tool for emotional regulation. I knew I was onto something here.

From a clinical perspective, bibliotherapy offers adolescents a profound sense of redemption and hope as they navigate the often-tumultuous transitions that life throws their way. This pivotal stage is marked by a series of profound shifts in identity, autonomy, and relationships, creating a fertile ground for emotional upheaval and uncertainty. Through the pages of a well-chosen book, teenagers discover that redemption and hope are attainable, and essential, components of their growth journey.

BIBLIOTHERAPY WITH ELDERS

When working with older adults, it's crucial to honor the diverse chapters of their life stories to support them in crafting the next one. Literature becomes a unique tool to explore these life stories, fostering healing and growth as we age. This aligns with Erikson's notion of leaving a lasting impact in the seventh stage of psychosocial development, where we seek to be valuable, accomplish goals, and contribute to society. Success at this stage means taking pride in our achievements and our relationships, while failure can lead to feelings of disconnection and unfulfillment. Literature serves as a mirror reflecting our present selves, as well as our ever-evolving selves.

In this next case study, we'll explore the meaningful impact of using literature for healing, understanding, and personal growth. Through the story of Mrs. Edith, a brave sixty-four-year-old woman navigating the challenges of widowhood, we witness how books can be a powerful tool for self-discovery, even in later stages of life. Mrs. E.'s unique journey revolves around her changing sexuality, addressing issues like menopause, societal expectations, and the pursuit of pleasure. We'll see how she draws inspiration from the concept of pleasure activism, which emphasizes joy, desire, and self-care as vital aspects of well-being. This case study showcases the accessible and universal healing potential of bibliotherapy, demonstrating its ability to guide readers in embracing our identities and desires, regardless of age or life experiences.

CASE STUDY:
SOULFUL LIBERATION:
NAVIGATING PLEASURE, GROWTH, AND HEALING
THROUGH BIBLIOTHERAPY IN LATER LIFE

When I first met Mrs. Edith, a sixty-four-year-old African American woman who was mourning the loss of her husband of forty years, I was struck by her unique approach to wanting to work with me. Mrs. E (she liked when I shortened her name because it made her feel "fly," ha ha) surprised me by requesting a bibliotherapy session focused on her sexuality, a request not often encountered in my practice, particularly with older adults. This request immediately piqued my curiosity, and I became eager to understand more about Mrs. E's specific needs and objectives regarding literature-based therapy.

She candidly shared her life experiences with me, including her recent retirement from her nursing career, her deeply loving marriage, her choice not to have children, and her late husband's involvement in the kink community before their marriage, to which he then introduced her. She emphasized the profound importance of addressing issues related to her shifting sense of sexuality and the hormonal changes she was undergoing, which would play a central role in our therapeutic journey together.

Mrs. E sought bibliotherapy as a means of reconnecting to her body and grief healing after the loss of her late husband. She described the myriad challenges many women face as they navigate the complex terrain of adjusting to a new life stage. Like countless others, she has experienced the profound shifts that come with age, including the natural process of menopause. This transformative phase, marked by hormonal changes, brought about various physical and emotional adjustments that affected her relationship to her body and sexuality. Mrs. E explained that she was reading more erotica than she ever had and wondered what this meant about her unique desires.

Mrs. E's candid exploration of these changes, a topic often shrouded in silence for my other Black femme clients, made it possible for us to normalize her experiences. She was grappling with shifts in her sexuality and her quest to rediscover pleasure and intimacy as she embraced her new chapter. She wanted to reduce her sense of shame for still wanting to be seen as a sexual being despite growing older.

Mrs. E had recently expressed a desire to reconnect with her sexual self and embrace her authentic needs after years of social pressure to present a specific way as a heterosexual, cisgender, married Black woman. She believed that her past experiences in the kink community her late husband had introduced her to had connected her profoundly to her fantasies and desires, which had since become obscured after his passing. (A kink community is a social network of individuals who share an interest in nontraditional sexual practices or preferences, often involving BDSM (bondage, discipline, dominance, submission, sadism, and masochism) activities. These communities provide a supportive environment for exploring and discussing diverse sexual desires, identities, and lifestyles.) I recognized that Mrs. E's journey toward healing and self-discovery could be enriched by the principles of pleasure activism.

Pleasure activism, described by writer/activist adrienne maree brown, is a transformative approach that centers joy, pleasure, and desire as essential components of activism and personal well-being. Pleasure activism challenges the dominant narratives that often associate activism solely with struggle and sacrifice. Instead, pleasure activism recognizes that the pursuit of pleasure is not a selfish endeavor but an integral part of social justice work. It encourages individuals to tap into their desires and sensual energy as sources of empowerment.

Through pleasure activism, people learn to prioritize self-care, self-love, and joy, recognizing that these elements are essential for their mental and emotional health. They are also vital for sustaining and strengthening movements for social change, even the personal movement of reclaiming one's own pleasure. In essence, pleasure activism seeks to create a world where pleasure and justice coexist, allowing individuals to live authentically and embrace their desires while actively working toward a more equitable and inclusive society. As an elder, Mrs. E truly enjoyed reading brown's words and considering her unique challenges through this philosophy of reclamation.

To address Mrs. E's unique needs, we embarked on a bibliotherapeutic journey that also included the book *Sensual Faith: The Art of Coming Home to Your Body* by Lyvonne Briggs. In *Sensual Faith*, Briggs invites women to embrace a healthier perspective on spirituality and sexuality, emphasizing pleasure over shame. She explains the notion that religious spaces have historically excluded the body, advocating for radical self-hospitality as the remedy. I knew that this book prescription would encourage Mrs. E to accept her body, nurture her intuition, prioritize pleasure, and practice sumptuous self-care on her journey to reclaim her sexuality. For Mrs. E, this was less about the act of sex and more about returning to herself from an embodied place that honored her changes while exploring new ways of being sensual. *Sensual Faith* served as a catalyst for exploring the concept of pleasure activism.

As Mrs. E immersed herself in the book, she resonated with the author's journey toward self-acceptance and sensual awakening. The book provided a safe space for her to explore her desires, experiences, and emotions. Through discussions and reflections inspired by the book, Mrs. E embraced her sensual energy and recognized its significance in her life. We worked to reframe inherited false narratives to guide our therapeutic journey, allowing her to integrate her past kink-community experiences into her broader life narrative.

Here is one quote that deeply resonated with Mrs. E from the text:

From a young age, we as Black, female children were hyper-sexualized and treated as if we were older than we actually were. A study on the adultification of Black girls conducted by Georgetown Law's Center on Poverty and Inequality found that adults viewed Black girls as young as five (5!) as needing "less nurturing, protection, support, and comfort than white girls of the same age." With teachers, pastors, coaches, and other caregivers believing these falsehoods, it's no wonder our childhoods were like vapor in the wind. We spent our years dodging racists, sexists, *and* pedophiles. That's not what childhood is supposed to be about. Some of us are blaming ourselves for things that simply weren't our fault. And if we cannot forgive ourselves for something we didn't do, we end up perpetually stuck.

After reading *Sensual Faith*, Mrs. E made important connections between her disconnection from her body and her internalized shame about having any desire to pursue pleasure at her age in the first place. Reading Briggs' book, Mrs. E was reminded that her husband was her first love. He was the first man who ever made her feel at home in her body. The first partner who introduced her to the kink community, a community that became found family when she moved to New York and left behind her life in South Carolina. Through our bibliotherapy journey, Mrs. E was reminded that pleasure is her birthright and something she deserves to feel again at any age and every stage of life. She learned to prioritize self-care practices that promoted her well-being and self-love, reigniting her sense of joy and vitality.

Over the course of our work together, Mrs. E experienced a profound transformation that supported her in releasing body shame. In *The Body Is Not an Apology*, author Sonya Renee Taylor reminds us:

> Across the landscapes of our existence we see [body shame's] ravages everywhere and feel acutely conscious of all the glorious chances we have not taken because of it. We ache for all the opportunities we ignored. Splattered before us like bugs on the windshield of life are all the ways we have shrunk the full expression of ourselves because we have been convinced that our bodies and therefore our very beings are deficient. We can also see how our inability to get out of our shame story amplifies our feelings of inadequacy. Our presumed failure at attaining some body-love nirvana becomes just another source of shame.

Mrs. E not only reconnected with her sexual energy—she also released her shame story and gained a newfound sense of self-worth and empowerment. The grief healing came from her newfound acceptance of herself and how her sexuality could look in this season of her life. Embracing the changes she was experiencing, she viewed herself as constantly evolving and no longer lacking.

Mrs. E's journey exemplifies the power of bibliotherapy to facilitate healing and personal acceptance across the lifespan. It showcases how literature, in conjunction with therapeutic guidance, can empower individuals to embrace their unique identities, tap into their desires, and embark on a path toward self-discovery and self-love. Her story demonstrates that regardless of one's age or life experiences, the healing potential of bibliotherapy remains boundless.

Mrs. E's bibliotherapeutic journey also highlights the profound impact of literature on navigating the complexities of sexuality and grief and invites us to consider how literature can be a guiding force through various rites of passage in life. As we progress through different phases of adulthood, literature provides a reflective mirror that allows us to explore and make sense of our evolving identities. In the absence of formal rites of passage, which are often culturally defined, literature becomes a source of wisdom, offering narratives that resonate with the nuances of our personal evolutions.

In essence, literature becomes a companion in the journey toward self-discovery at every age, helping readers to contextualize our experiences and find meaning in the twists and turns of life. Whether it's the challenges of menopause, the complexities of identity, or the pursuit of pleasure, literature serves as a nonjudgmental guide, offering diverse perspectives and stories that validate our experiences on a deeply personal level. Mrs. E's story illustrates how, through literature, we each can navigate the uncharted territories of our lives, finding inspiration, understanding, and a sense of connection that transcends the limitations of formal rites of passage.

NARRATIVES THAT RESONATE WITH PERSONAL TRANSFORMATION

Here are just a few examples of literature that contain themes of personal transformation and important rites of passage that mark our growth, from one life phase or stage to the next:

The Alchemist by Paulo Coelho: This allegorical novel tells the story of Santiago, a shepherd boy, on his quest for the fulfillment of his dreams. The narrative is a metaphorical journey that explores the transformative power of following one's heart.

Becoming by Michelle Obama: In her memoir, the former First Lady reflects on her life, from childhood to the White House, highlighting the personal transformations that stand out most. The narrative delves into identity, purpose, and the evolution of self, never shying away from the intersectionality of her experiences as a Black woman. Michelle Obama's memoir, *Becoming*, offers a profound reflection on identity, purpose, and personal growth. What makes the intersectionality in her memoir so special is how it intertwines her roles as a Black woman, a daughter, a wife, a mother, and a First Lady—all while navigating spaces that are predominantly white and male-dominated. Michelle's experiences as a Black woman in America provide readers with a deeply nuanced perspective on systemic inequality, as well as the strength and resilience required to rise above it.

Through her storytelling, Obama showcases how her racial and gender identity shaped her journey, while also inviting readers to reflect on how their own intersectional identities influence their life experiences. Her openness about dealing with issues like imposter syndrome, being scrutinized for her physical appearance, and being underestimated, even when occupying a role as powerful as First Lady, creates a connection to the lived experiences of many women of color. By sharing her vulnerabilities alongside her triumphs, she challenges stereotypes and celebrates the fullness of Black womanhood.

This intersectionality component is also vital because Michelle Obama's life story transcends a singular narrative. She gives voice to both the personal and political, reflecting on the broader implications of what it means to be a Black woman at the highest levels of public life while maintaining her authentic self. In doing so, she not only celebrates the beauty of Black identity but also invites readers of all backgrounds to find strength in embracing their unique selves.

The Kite Runner by Khaled Hosseini: This novel explores the complexities of friendship, betrayal, and redemption. The characters undergo significant transformations as they grapple with guilt, forgiveness, and the impact of their past actions. The story also details how immigrants' unique migration stories can both perpetuate trauma and catalyze culturally sensitive modes of healing.

Their Eyes Were Watching God by Zora Neale Hurston: This classic novel follows the journey of Janie Crawford as she navigates love, loss, and self-discovery in the early twentieth century. Hurston's narrative explores Janie's quest for independence and personal fulfillment, making it a powerful portrayal of a woman's transformation in a time that marked a number of social and political convergences.

The Color Purple by Alice Walker: In this Pulitzer Prize–winning novel, Walker tells the story of Celie, an African American woman living in the early twentieth century who overcomes adversity and abuse to find her voice and identity. The narrative explores themes of found family, self-love, Blackness, and queer identity, offering a compelling exploration of how we might rewrite our life stories to find purpose in the unlikeliest places.

Whether in the form of novels, memoirs, or poetry, literature provides a mirror to our own experiences, a window into diverse perspectives, and a doorway to empathy. In times of joy or sorrow, triumph and tribulation, the written word becomes a steadfast ally, guiding us through the ebbs and flows of our life journey. Although the path from infancy to elderhood is hardly linear and is shaped by many tributaries that flow into the same river, we can hold books up as valuable guides when it comes to initiating us into rites of passage that emphasize both our autonomy and our interconnectedness.

BIBLIOTHERAPEUTIC REFLECTION:

Consider the following questions to explore how books have played a role in normalizing your experiences and shedding false shame:

1. Recall a book or story that enabled you to feel a deep sense of identification with the characters or themes during a time in your life when you were being initiated into a new stage or phase (e.g., adolescence, young adulthood, motherhood, elderhood, etc.). How did this story help normalize aspects of your life and make you feel less alone in your struggles?

2. The process of getting older and wiser is a process of stepping into our authenticity, feeling more comfortable in our skin, and exercising courage in small and large ways. Reflect on books and stories that addressed taboos or stigmatized topics, providing a platform for open discussion and reflection. How did these narratives contribute to breaking the silence around certain issues, allowing you to confront and challenge social norms or personal misconceptions? What were the ripple effects on the people in your life?

3. Think about a book or story that inspired a period of immense growth and liberation by helping you to challenge limiting beliefs or expectations (familial, social, cultural, national, etc.). How did the characters' journey influence your mindset and help you shed false shame associated with certain aspects of your identity or experiences? Did your concept of your identity transform in the process? How?

CONCLUSION
EMBRACING THE GENTLE PATH

Accept yourself. Find yourself. Be kind to yourself, and then find others to share the feeling. You belong to you. Like ocean glass, you are formed by the world around you. You belong to the community of humans, plants, and animals that share this planet. Allow everything that comes your way, like the wind and waves that shape glass to a frosted, polished surface, to shape and reshape your heart until you become a fuller, richer, more alive expression of you.

—VALERIE BROWN, *Hope Leans Forward: Braving Your Way Toward Simplicity, Awakening, and Peace*

In the cozy embrace of a sunlit room, a plush armchair awaits your arrival. As you settle into its comforting contours, your fingers gently caress the pages of a well-loved book, feeling the slightly textured surface beneath your touch. You inhale the faint scent of ink and paper, a subtle reminder of the countless stories that have come before this one. The weight of the book in your hands is substantial, grounding you in the present moment.

Opening the book, you embark on a multisensory journey. As your eyes traverse the words on the pages, they become windows into vivid worlds, and you're transported to places unknown. You hear the characters' voices in your mind, their dialogues resonating like soft whispers or thundering declarations. With each turn of the page, a symphony of emotions begins to play, the rising crescendos of joy, heartache, and suspense reverberating within you.

Time seems to stand still as you lose yourself in the narrative. The tactile sensation of the paper beneath your fingertips anchors you while the words dance like ethereal melodies in your thoughts. You taste the bittersweet tears of the protagonist's journey, the warmth of their triumphs, and the tang of their challenges. Your emotions swell and ebb, mirroring the characters' experiences, forging an empathetic connection that transcends the boundaries of the book.

The act of reading becomes a sanctuary, a place of solace and self-discovery. It is a gentle therapeutic journey, guiding you through the labyrinth of your emotions, much like the characters navigating their own destinies. With each chapter, you peel back the layers of your psyche—finding resonance, understanding, and healing in the stories that unfold.

As a therapist, I invite you to immerse yourself in the pleasurable nature of reading to ground you in the present moment, to allow the written word to touch your senses, your emotions, and your soul. Through literature, we unlock the power of introspection, empathy, and catharsis, enabling profound healing and self-transformation. So, continue to embrace the tactile, auditory, and emotional richness of reading, for within these pages lies the potential for growth, insight, and the soothing balm of self-discovery.

MAKING READING FUN AGAIN

Reading should be fun, but for many children, young people, and adults alike, the pressures of schooling make it feel like a difficult task. When I work with young people who struggle with reading and reading comprehension, my goal is always to affirm that they, too, can access joy in the power of stories. For centuries, long before any of us were born, indigenous tradition and oral storytelling were our primary ways of relating and sharing our history throughout the generations.

Stories are always being told, and they will always be told. This is a skill that helps us connect to our truths and to each other. It is a deeply personal way to access language that is in our blood.

No one should ever be made to feel that they cannot access the beauty of stories, especially their own, because of a struggle to read or write. We always have access to our truth deep inside of us, and the job of the teacher, the leader, and the bibliotherapist is to guide the client through the process of identifying exactly what story needs telling and how to go about sharing it. For many youths, music is an entry point to storytelling. For others, it's an exercise in sharpening their listening skills and considering the many stories being told daily around them: the sound of a loved one on the phone in the kitchen, the homeless man preaching on the corner of the block, the way the birds tweet and hum from inside the comfort of tree branches. Stories are always being told. We just have to take the time to listen.

According to the Scholastic *Kids & Family Reading Report*, 89 percent of kids say their favorite books are the ones they picked out themselves. When children have the freedom to choose their own books, it often leads to a greater sense of engagement and enjoyment in reading. Allowing children to select their books enables them to explore subjects, genres, and stories that align with their personal interests. When kids are drawn to books that appeal to them, they are more likely to be motivated to read and have a positive reading experience. Giving children agency to choose their books also promotes a sense of ownership and autonomy over their reading choices, boosting their intrinsic motivation to read. Balancing personal choice with guided reading recommendations can help create a well-rounded reading experience and serve as a protective factor against literacy trauma.

For me personally, bibliotherapy and creative arts therapies provide an accessible and holistic way to decolonize therapy, access healing, and make the work of repair stimulating and cathartic. When I think about decolonizing therapy, a core value comes to mind: recognizing the importance of centering the voices, experiences, and knowledge of individuals and communities who have historically been marginalized or excluded from mainstream therapeutic practices. Decolonizing therapy questions and challenges dominant narratives and norms that shape therapeutic theories and practices (even the ones I mention in this book). It critiques the universalization of Western psychological frameworks and encourages the exploration of alternative cultural and indigenous healing practices.

Decolonizing therapy emphasizes cultural responsiveness and cultural humility. It requires that, as therapists, we engage in ongoing self-reflection, education, and examination of our biases and assumptions. Approaches that honor self-healing practice and build on the strengths of our clients decenter the therapist and center the client as the expert on their own lives. We honor our clients' experiences by acknowledging and addressing the intergenerational impacts of colonialism, historical trauma, and systemic oppression. Cultivating and incorporating a love of literature into healing practice integrates an approach that promotes healing, empowerment, collaboration, and shared decision-making and shifts the power dynamic between therapist and client by encouraging their active participation in the therapeutic process. Some of my most successful bibliotherapy sessions have been using texts my clients recommend to me and not the other way around.

In *Pleasure Activism*, adrienne maree brown writes about those who taught her to center her pleasure in life and say yes to herself. Among the impactful voices she mentions are several women of color, such as Octavia Butler, Audre Lorde, and Toni Cade Bambara. The work of writers like Anaïs Nin, Alice Walker, Andrea Dworkin, and Erica Jong taught her what sex could be and how to become sexually liberated outside of a framework that seeks to serve men. She speaks to the truth that many of us have come to distrust our inherent power and knowledge, the wisdom that resides in our bones. When we embrace self-connection, we remind ourselves and our bodies of our capacity for feeling. More importantly, we remind ourselves how it feels to feel good and how much we deserve to feel the goodness of life. *Pleasure Activism* was one of the first books that helped me integrate the idea that joy, pleasure, and celebration are essential components of transformative social change and healing.

As a bibliophile and therapist, my love of reading and the incorporation of literature into healing practice are my activism. It's double the reward because I get to work with those for whom reading brings pleasure just as much as it does for me. Engaging in activities that bring pleasure and joy allows us to reclaim agency over our lives. We don't have to choose between our books or our desire to seek therapy; we can do both. In contexts where we might feel disempowered, marginalized, or oppressed, pleasure activism empowers us to assert our desires and preferences, fostering a sense of autonomy and control in the therapy room and beyond.

I love that my clients enjoy speaking with me about their fictional crushes and the parts of themselves they are afraid to let other people see—parts that are allowed to come out and play, simply be, and imagined freely during pleasure reading. Pleasure activism includes the communal experiences we create for ourselves as literature lovers, creating spaces for people to come together, share our challenges and our victories, and build supportive communities. These connections are healing, as they provide a sense of belonging and solidarity. These connections are what make healing possible—and evidence-based or not, we do not owe anyone an explanation for what has gotten us over.

We are here. We are still here. We will be here. With our ever-growing TBR (to-be-read) lists and all our bookish opinions and our book friends, too. When we are reading, we are healing. When we are reading, we are witnessing and allowing our feelings to be honored and witnessed, too.

BIBLIOTHERAPEUTIC REFLECTION

Affirm to yourself out loud:

I am a reader.
I am a storyteller.
I am always learning.
I am forever evolving.

I do not have to be anyone or anything other than who I am today.
My story matters.
My story is still being written.
I give myself permission to write, read, and revise.

AFTERWORD

In the spirit of transparency, I am a bibliotherapy enthusiast, but more specifically, a Literapy NYC and Emely Rumble enthusiast. I had been engaging with bibliotherapy for years, both personally and professionally, without knowing that it was a thing. To me, the exercise of engaging with print as a means of interrogation and reflection was simply book medicine, or rather, *word medicine.*

And then I came across Emely's work, and she opened my eyes and gave my medicine a name. Much like the elder who shares a salve or tincture and all of the ways to preserve and use the herbs the gardener is already planting or foraging, Emely's work came into my life and expanded my lens and the impact of what I already was using. She was and is my biblio-apotherapist. An alchemist. Since then, I have been sold on this modality, both in my studies and my practice. And though I have learned much about its history, its uses, and the work of other practitioners and teachers, I always come back to my well, which is Emely's wisdom and unparalleled expertise on the topic. For me, bibliotherapy and Emely are almost interchangeable terms. This is her zone of genius.

When I was invited to read her book, the very first thing that moved me (outside of, well, "This is Emely's work") was the title. I mean, Emely. Literapy NYC. Bibliotherapy? Why, yes, sign me up! And then, these three very specific words: *in the Bronx.* Cue Mama Tina's voice: *What's Bronx got to do with it?* My interest was additionally piqued.

Choosing a name that potentially disengages or even alienates potential new readers (a.k.a. buyers) does not come without a cost and risk. In the context of capitalism, more potential new readers means potential dollars, and more is, well, *more*. As someone who has written a book whose title leads with naming a very specific demographic/space, I was immediately vested in the intentionality of the name.

There's a lot of context contained in the name of this specific borough: ***The Bronx. Poor. Black. Latinx. Immigrant. Brown. Illiterate. Blue Collar. Busy. Loud. Broken.*** As I read the title, every one of those things was called in, named, centered. I wanted to read more. Humanity-centering systems understand that liberation happens in the margin and serving the margin is the way we ensure that all humanity is served.

By now, you've read the book. For all intents and purposes, you know, this book could have very well been titled something along the lines of *The Case for Bibliotherapy*, to cast a wider net. Certainly, the contents of each page and its frameworks, case studies, and reflective questions make it a suitable study text for all students, as well as conventional and nontraditional mental health professionals. Emely has carved herself a place in all bibliotherapy studies with this book. It is a reference book. A resource. And relevant to every demographic. And still, the book's title is *Bibliotherapy in the Bronx*.

If we pause to think about it, Emely has already prescribed us a dose of bibliotherapy before even going into the content. The title is the invitation to interrogate. As we accept the invitation, the words on each chapter are the prize. Quoting her words from inside the book: **"You can still experience the immense power of words as witnesses, regardless of where you come from and what letters you might have after your name."**

I wasn't ten pages into the book when I paused and said to myself, "Oh, Emely. Look at what you did, sis—they gotta get through the title to get to *this*? Snap, snap."

The idea of bibliotherapy, a therapeutic modality that centers literacy, happening in a place normally not associated with either mental wellness or literacy has to be the very thing that makes you reach for the book. Her bookshake brings all the boys (and girls and nonbinary folx) to the yard, and she willingly teaches us, but our admission fee is our curiosity. The shedding of our bias and our willingness to reject or be attracted to a book that centers a marginalized place and communities.

Poor Black and Brown people read. They write. They feel. They suffer. They endure. They seek healing. They heal. They care. They commune. They do and are all the things the world tells you they are not and don't do. We are. We do. The Bronx. Birthplace of hip-hop. Seriously, what more bibliotherapy-ish place than the Bronx? Of course, *Bibliotherapy in the Bronx*. You must be this tall (aware) to enjoy this ride!

Among my favorite parts of the book is the imagery of Emely reading Psalm 23 at her grandmother's funeral and naming this act bibliotherapy. I also appreciate the vulnerable share that she—who, for so many, myself included, is the voice and face of bibliotherapy—is not yet officially "credentialed" in this modality. She could have omitted that disclosure. Truly, she could have. In a world of social media, where perception is reality, her expertise would have carried the perception. And yet, she made room with those two shares: a devastated teen Emely and a professional, "uncredentialed" bibliotherapist Emely, for us to see ourselves in this space. And we are better for it.

To quote her own words, her inspiration for writing the book was "to emphasize that bibliotherapy transcends conventional notions of qualification, and its impact is felt by all, irrespective of their educational background or formal credentials." It is clear to me that the comprehensive nature of the book is very much meant to support both professionals and students in this field, as well as the many people who, in a myriad of spaces, much like the Bronx, must employ a form of self-didacticism to have access to therapeutic modalities. So often, this is the reality of marginalized folks, gatekept out of medical, education, or credentialing systems. In this light, many of us must independently seek out, learn, and access resources in order to survive. If this was the inspiration, we rejoice in its manifestation. Years from now, we will read many more books, in many more places, with many more case studies and stories, of people who read *Bibliotherapy in the Bronx* and were compelled to study, practice, and heal through bibliotherapy. This much I know.

NIKOLAI PIZARRO
Author of *Ring the Alarm: The Hope of Black and Brown Communities: A Zero to Five Parenting Guide for Low Income Black and Latino Caregivers*

ACKNOWLEDGMENTS

I am deeply grateful to Rebekah Borucki, founder and president of Row House Publishing, for not only seeing my vision for this book but also honoring and championing it. Your belief in this project has been a cornerstone of its success.

To my editor, Nirmala Nataraj, who was like a midwife to me during the writing process: your clarity, compassion, and spiritual might helped transform my vision into a reality. I hope this book supports many readers and bibliotherapists along the way.

To every mentor and guide who has nurtured my path to this day, there are too many to name, and I fear missing some important names, but you know who you are. Your wisdom and support have been invaluable. I will never forget you and the impact you've had on my life's journey.

I want to specifically thank my mother, Diane Velez, for giving me life and enduring so much so that my life could be possible. To my grandmother, Rosa Jimenez, thank you for being a guiding light and force in my life in every realm.

My heartfelt gratitude goes to my mentors: Davita Westbrook, Rosemary Jackson, Fred Jackson, Kenya Neabar, Marcus Neabar, Val Bryan, Vincent Calenda, Ella Berthoud, Sherry Reiter, Pamela Nomura, Mary Caminiti, Carolyn Mangiafico, and Jeanette Luciano.

To my best friend and sister for life, Alexis Suib, you are one of a kind. I love you.

To God(dess), my guides, and my ancestors, known and unknown, for an abundance of love, provision, and protection that cannot be quantified. I honor you.

Special thanks to my beta readers. To Seanathan Polidore, for keeping me grounded in my authenticity and reminding me to stay true to the communities this book is for. To my dear late friend Natasha Anderson, without whom this book would not have been completed. There isn't a day that goes by that I do not hear her voice in my head, reminding me to be kind to myself and to always lead with self-compassion as a guide. May her husband and children always know how much they meant to her. I will never forget her.

I also want to thank the Black feminist writers who have directly influenced my reading practice, spiritual practice, and light work in this world. These present-day writers tirelessly build on the work of our literary greats and contribute significantly to literature, social justice, and feminist theory, shaping the discourse on race, gender, and identity, past and present. These include, but are not limited to, Imani Perry, Ruha Benjamin, Brittney Cooper, Roxane Gay, Jenn M. Jackson, Yaba Blay, Bettina Love, EbonyJanice Moore, adrienne maree brown, Alexis Pauline Gumbs, and Loren Cahill. Your work has illuminated my path and inspired me profoundly.

To readers worldwide: Thank you for all the heart work you put into sharing your love of books and building care networks within literary communities. Always keep reading.

BIBLIOGRAPHY

Acevedo, Elizabeth. *The Poet X*. New York: HarperCollins, 2018.

Alexander, Kwame. *Kwame Alexander's Free Write: A Poetry Notebook*. Naperville: Sourcebooks Wonderland, 2023.

American Library Association. Library War Service. Ann Arbor: University of Michigan Library, 1920.

Angelou, Maya. *I Know Why the Caged Bird Sings*. 1969. Reprint, New York: Random House, 2010.

Arango, Andrea Beatriz. *Iveliz Explains It All*. Washington, DC: National Geographic Books, 2022.

"Banned Books | Penguin Random House." *Penguin Random House*. Accessed September 19, 2024. www.penguinrandomhouse.com/ banned-books/.

Belafonte, Harry, and Michael Shnayerson. *My Song: A Memoir*. New York: Alfred A. Knopf, 2011.

Black, Daniel. *The Coming*. New York: St. Martin's Press, 2015.

"Books & More - Carnegie Library of Pittsburgh." *Carnegie Library of Pittsburgh*, September 5, 2024. Accessed September 19, 2024. www .carnegielibrary.org/books-media/.

Browne, Anthony. *Hansel and Gretel*. London: Walker Books, 2008.

Callender, Kacen. *Felix Ever After*. New York: HarperCollins, 2020.

Cisneros, Sandra. *The House on Mango Street*. New York: Vintage Books, 1991.

Clear, James. *Atomic Habits: An Easy & Proven Way to Build Good Habits & Break Bad Ones*. New York: Avery, 2018.

Coelho, Paulo. *The Alchemist*. 2006. Reprint, New York: HarperCollins, 2006.

DeGruy, Joy. *Post Traumatic Slave Syndrome*. New York: HarperCollins, 2017.

der Weduwen, Arthur, and Andrew Pettegree. *The Library: A Fragile History*. London: Profile Books, 2021.

Diuguid, Bradley. "Sadie Peterson Delaney and the Work of Bibliotherapy." *Poughkeepsie Public Library District*. Accessed August 5, 2020. poklib.org/sadie-peterson-delaney-and-the-work-of-bibliotherapy/.

electricliterature. "Books as Medicine: A Conversation with Sandra Cisneros." *Electric Literature*, November 2, 2015. Accessed August 5, 2020. electricliterature.com/books-as-medicine-a-conversation-with-sandra-cisneros/.

Fighting Words. HBO Max. Accessed September 30, 2024. https://www.hbo.com/movies/aida-rodriguez-fighting-words.

Fisher, Antwone Q., and Mim E. Rivas. *Finding Fish*. New York: HarperCollins, 2009.

Forgan, James W. "Using Bibliotherapy to Teach Problem Solving." *Intervention in School and Clinic* 38, no. 2 (November 2002): 75–82. https://doi.org/10.1177/10534512020380020201.

Hynes, Arleen McCarty, and Mary Hynes-Berry. *Biblio/Poetry Therapy: The Interactive Process: A Handbook*. St. Cloud: North Star Press of St. Cloud, 2012.

Jack, S. J., and K. R. Ronan. "Bibliotherapy: Practice and Research." *School Psychology International* 29, no. 2 (2008): 161–182. https://doi.org/10.1177/0143034308090058.

Kaur, Rupi. *Healing through Words*. 2022.

"Kids & Family Reading Report - Scholastic." Scholastic.com. Accessed September 30, 2024. https://www.scholastic.com/content/dam/ KFRR/PastReports/KFRR2017_6th.pdf.

Laymon, Kiese. *Long Division*. New York: Simon & Schuster, 2021.

Leahey, Thomas H. "The Mythical Revolutions of American Psychology." *American Psychologist* 47, no. 2 (1992): 308–318. https:// doi.org/10.1037//0003-066x.47.2.308.

Leilani, Raven. *Luster*. New York: Farrar, Strauss, and Giroux, 2020.

McCoy, Henrika, and Cassandra McKay. "Preparing Social Workers to Identify and Integrate Culturally Affirming Bibliotherapy into Treatment." *Social Work Education* 25, no. 7 (October 2006): 680– 693. https://doi.org/10.1080/02615470600905895.

Mullan, Jennifer. *Decolonizing Therapy: Oppression, Historical Trauma, and Politicizing Your Practice*. New York: W. W. Norton, 2023.

Nas. "It Ain't Hard to Tell." Illmatic. Produced by DJ Premier. 1993.

Nikki Giovanni and the New York Community Choir. Truth Is On Its Way. Right On Records, n.d.

Obama, Michelle. *Becoming*. New York: Crown, 2018.

Orlean, Susan. *The Library Book*. New York: Simon & Schuster, 2019.

Psalm 23. Grand Rapids, MI: Zondervan, 2008.

Rich, Adrienne. "Diving into the Wreck." *Poets.org*, May 15, 2019. https://poets.org/poem/diving-wreck.

Rodriguez, Aida. *Legitimate Kid*. New York: HarperCollins, 2023.

Ryan, Pam Muñoz. *Esperanza Rising*. 2000. Reprint, New York: Scholastic Press, 2000.

Sadie P. Delaney papers. Schomburg Center for Research in Black Culture, The New York Public Library.

Shange, Ntozake. *For Colored Girls Who Have Considered Suicide When the Rainbow Is Enuf*. Reprint Edition. New York: Scribner, 1997.

Smith, Katisha. "13 Pioneering Black American Librarians You Oughta Know." *BOOK RIOT*, May 8, 2020. Accessed October 17, 2020. https://bookriot.com/pioneering-black-american-librarians/.

"SRRT Resolutions 1976: Resolution on Racism and Sexism Awareness." American Library Association. September 6, 2019. Accessed September 30, 2024. https://www.ala.org/rt/srrt-resolutions-1976 -resolution-racism-and-sexism-awareness.

Stand Up and Shout: Songs From A Philly High School. US: Discovery Global Music Documentaries, 2023.

Taylor, Sonya Renee. *The Body Is Not an Apology*. Oakland: Berrett-Koehler Publishers, 2018.

Tyson, Edgar H. "Hip Hop Therapy: An Exploratory Study of a Rap Music Intervention with At-Risk and Delinquent Youth." *Journal of Poetry Therapy* 15, no. 3 (2002): 131–144.

Walker, Alice. *The Color Purple*. New York: Penguin Books, 2019.

INDEX

ABOUT THE AUTHOR

EMELY RUMBLE, LCSW, is a distinguished licensed clinical social worker, school social worker, and seasoned biblio/psychotherapist with more than fourteen years of professional experience. Committed to making mental health services more accessible, Emely specializes in the transformative practice of bibliotherapy.

Emely is passionate about advocating for the integration of creative arts in psychotherapy, mental well-being, and self-improvement. She champions the social model of disability and embraces a neurodiversity-affirming therapeutic approach. Emely's work has been featured in respected publications such as *Parents* magazine, *School Library Journal*, *Dazed* magazine, and *Success* magazine, by The Bronx Is Reading, and on BronxNet news.

Having earned her undergraduate degree from Mount Holyoke College and completed her social work degree at Smith College School for Social Work, Emely currently resides in Western Massachusetts with her family.

Emely shares her expertise beyond traditional avenues through @Literapy_NYC, her dedicated platform on social media, where she provides valuable educational content.